MW01014138

NINE MAGIC SECRETS
OF LONG LIFE

Also by Mr. Hill

HOW TO THINK LIKE A MILLIONAIRE AND GET RICH

NINE MAGIC
SECRETS
OF LONG LIFE

Howard E. Hill

Parker Publishing Company, Inc.
West Nyack, N.Y.

© 1979 *by*

Parker Publishing Company, Inc.

West Nyack, New York

All rights reserved. No part of this
book may be reproduced in any form or
by any means, without permission in
writing from the publisher.

This book is a reference work based on research by the
author. The opinions expressed herein are not necessarily
those of or endorsed by the publisher. The directions stated
in this book are in no way to be considered as a substitute for
consultation with a duly licensed doctor.

Library of Congress Cataloging in Publication Data

Hill, Howard E
  Nine magic secrets of long life.

  Includes index.
  1. Health. 2. Longevity. I. Title.
RA776.5.H47   613   78-27393
ISBN 0-13-622548-9

Printed in the United States of America

Dedicated to
Hattie Yearian Ives
My wonderful Mother-in-law
Who almost made it
to the century mark

WHAT THIS BOOK WILL
DO FOR YOU

When a man or woman first sets about the exciting venture of extending his span of years, the principal aim and intent should be to delay *physical maturity as long as possible,* or to slow down the aging process.

To accomplish this happy objective, I have studied and researched the field for the past thirty years — always seeking the simplest and least complicated methods that I could find, with special consideration given to those plans and programs closest to the elementary *Laws of Nature.* What I have discovered I now reveal to you, certain substances and actions of proved merit that will help you delay the aging process in yourself. They are so little known to most people I call them "secrets," and their results are often so impressive they seem like magic. There are essentially nine of these "magic secrets," all of them simple, natural ways to extend your active, enjoyable years of life far beyond all expectations.

The time to wake up and live joyously is NOW!

When you first become aware of the fact that no one branch of the healing arts has all the answers — in spite of greatly exaggerated claims of infallibility — you will be on your way to a longer and more rewarding way of life.

There is not one single shred of evidence to prove that drugs, surgery, adjustments, massage, mind, prayer, breath, vibration, fifty-mile hikes, natural remedies, or diets of fruits and vegetables will heal all of the ills of mankind, but there is considerable evidence that there is a time and place for each of these practices.

In my search for truth about the secrets of long life, I studied every school of thought or healing practice, evaluated them, and appraised them strictly on their merits — and the resulting answers have been quite revealing.

In the beginning of time, it was quite normal for a man or woman well versed in the truths of Natural Law to live as long as one-hundred-and-fifty years. Even today, we often hear of persons reaching this *advanced* age in the so-called primitive areas. Actually, this *ripe old age* is not unusual, for it was written in the *genesis* of mankind that to attain this reward of life, one only had to read the open book of nature, and abide by the laws of being so clearly demonstrated for us by the Creator.

When you have made the NINE MAGIC SECRETS OF LONG LIFE a part of your daily living routine, you will have a good chance to achieve, and energize, a long and vibrant life expression.

Howard E. Hill

TABLE OF CONTENTS

11

NINE MAGIC SECRETS
OF LONG LIFE

1

THE EXCITING
PERSONAL DISCOVERY OF
NINE MAGIC HEALTH SECRETS

If you want to increase your expectation of a long life, there are certain natural principles you need to know. I discovered these secrets a number of years ago. Actually, these *nine magic secrets of long life* are not really "secrets" in the true sense of that word, but they might just as well be, for so few persons are really aware of them.

My search for these secrets began when my doctor told me I had developed an incurable physical ailment — *degenerative arthritis* — from which there was no hope of recovery! This ailment, I learned, had been brought on by my hectic years of modern living. Needless to say, I did not much like this grim pronouncement. I wanted to live! Suddenly I was confronted with the fact that I had to learn a whole new set of values if I wanted to survive.

At this time I was rarely free of excruciating pain, but life was precious to me, and I determined to do something about my problem at once. Although I am not a doctor, and have had no medical training, I began to undertake extensive research into healthful living. With my new-found knowledge, I was able to conquer the crippling illness myself. I regained my health through the discovery of the Nine Magic Secrets which I am shortly going to reveal to you.

MY FIRST DISCOVERY

Even before I found out about the Nine Magic Secrets, I discovered that my painful affliction was derived from careless habits of living, little or no attention to the quality of food that I was eating, and worst of all, eating too hurriedly, under pressure. Fast food snacks and convenience foods were high on my menu list. I learned that these foods were almost totally *devitalized*.

I continued my personal research, through endless hours of reading, of checking and cross-checking references, and seemingly countless days of interviewing well-known nutritionists, health food store operators, and lecturers on health improvement. I figured any or all of these might be helpful to me, at least in describing ways to lessen the pain I was going through.

At first my search was largely "trial and error," but gradually my investigating led me to certain basic natural laws. I found out more and more about vitamins, minerals and nutrients. As I learned, I applied what I had learned to my own living habits. I experimented with natural foods and beverages. Nine principles emerged as particularly important.

As a result of my studies and application of these nine principles, I have achieved complete recovery from my "incurable" illness, and I now have an expectation of many years of life.

A few years earlier, my intense interest in more successful living had become widely known, and inspired Dr. Greg Ziemer, formerly director of the Institute of Lifetime Learning, in Long Beach, California, to invite me to lead classes there. Members of my classes included members of the American Association of Retired Persons and the National Retired Teachers Association.

Most of the men and women who attended my classes and participated in discussions were past middle age, nearing retirement, or already retired, but they all had an intense desire to live a *long, healthy and active life.* Nearly everyone enrolled in my classes felt they had barely survived the rigors of poor nutrition, the pressure of modern patterns of living, and the urgencies of trying to survive in a highly competitive society.

GRACE V. TRIES THE "MAGIC SECRETS"

One instance I recall quite vividly was that of Grace V., who, by diligence and hard work, had been named head of the history department of her college prior to her retirement. She felt her struggle to achieve her position had left her weak, constantly fatigued, and without hope. Since other prescriptions and programs had failed to give this lady any relief, she decided to try the nine magic secrets. She applied all of these in an active program.

Within three weeks, Grace V. began to blossom forth as a "new woman." She began to seem younger right away. "It was nothing short of a miracle," she informed me during a class session.

Shortly afterward I learned that Grace V. was planning a round-the-world cruise in order to visit many of the notable and historic places she had been talking about in her history classes for so many years. She had planned this many years earlier, but had practically abandoned the venture because she feared she would never live through the experience. Now she looked forward to the cruise with great excitement.

The foregoing "case" is only one of dozens of heart-warming stories that came to my attention during the many years I lectured at the Institute. In nearly every instance, men and women who have given my program a fair trial have discovered that the *nine magic secrets* have opened up a whole new way of life, full of challenges and excitement for them. And I am my own best example. Today, years after my doctor pronounced my doom, I am living a full, active life which would be considered quite strenuous at times for a man of half my years, and I am loving every minute of my busy schedule.

THE VALUE OF MY GROUP

When I accepted the assignment from Dr. Ziemer to teach a class in Better Living, ten years ago, I had no idea that two years later I would be stricken with degenerative arthritis, an excruciatingly painful and debilitating experience. Poor health, of course, is hardly compatible with "better living." Many of the men and women in my class suffered from similar ailments. I was supposed to be the authority, but I was hard-pressed for answers to their health problems, when I was so obviously suffering myself. My own condition was all too obvious, and I could hardly conceal it from such an intelligent group of former teachers, a variety of professional people, and hardheaded business men and women.

My good doctor, an M.D. of some repute, could only prescribe expensive pain killers for what ailed me. To make matters worse, he informed me that I would never be able to walk again without the aid of an aluminum-frame "walker." To push myself around on that contraption the rest of my life was a condition I refused to accept.

Undaunted, I began to evaluate, with my class, all of the instruction I had previously been offering them. From the beginning it was quite plain that I had to take my group into my confidence. I challenged others in the group to try my new life plan along with me. I was fortunate enough to have three people in my group who accepted my challenge — a retired telephone company executive, a schoolteacher, and a very skeptical former head nurse of a major hospital who refused at the time to let her name be used in connection with what she termed "an experiment."

Because my interest in my own recovery was so great and demanding, I wanted some valid answers — fast. Within three weeks I had the beginnings of my new better living program, applying nine secrets of health, in sound working order. With my friends in the group, I applied what I had learned rigorously.

All of us had to make some changes in our lives. But we asked ourselves whether we wanted to go on suffering pain and living as handicapped persons, or did we want to regain our good health? It didn't take any of us long to answer that one.

I myself began to improve within a few days, and within three months I was once again living a normal life. Today — years later — I live a full, active life, even strenuous at times by ordinary standards.

SOME DRAMATIC RECOVERIES

During the years since I began revealing my findings about the Nine Magic Secrets to the hundreds of people who attended my lectures, I have seen some exceedingly remarkable recoveries. I'm happy to report a few of the most dramatic of these. For example, the former telephone company executive, who shuffled into class sessions with the aid of two stout canes, began to improve in a most miraculous fashion. He was 79 at the time he first came to my class. Now, several years later, he is amazingly spry and active for his age.

The retired teacher I mentioned earlier had once had to forsake her cherished music because of almost constant pain in her arms and hands. Now she found herself able to resume playing in a small "combo" that entertained in nearby clubs. She and her "combo" still accept engagements two or three times a week from all manner of groups.

But the story that amuses and gratifies me the most is the one about the retired head nurse from the biggest hospital in the area. At the age of 76 she was on the verge of being bedridden. This lady signed on for my lectures more as a way to pass the time than to learn anything of value, and she prepared to argue with me about my "kooky ideas" about nutrition.

In our earlier class sessions together, her questions were very searching, and heavily tinged with skepticism, but it wasn't long before she decided it was only fair to try out my better living program, using the Nine Magic Secrets. The results were startling. Within six weeks she was close to complete recovery, and two months later she was as close to normal activity as a person her age could be.

During the years since, I have known many persons who, like me, discovered the nine magic secrets — and this includes men and women of all backgrounds who are living healthier, happier lives because these secrets were revealed to them.

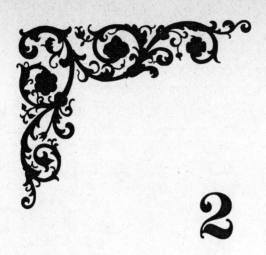

2

HOW TO USE GOOD FOOD
AS BUILDING BLOCKS
FOR A LONG LIFE

Before I begin discussing the Nine Magic Secrets, I want to establish a general understanding of the importance of good nutrition to your life. When you understand how to eat for good health, you have a good background for use of the Nine Magic Secrets.

Most people find it extremely difficult to remember the principles of sound nutrition in their daily lives. Unfortunately, at mealtime nearly everybody decides what to eat or not to eat entirely by taste, and they often choose to eat something pleasant tasting which is bad for them.

If you have been taught nutritional values, you often find

it difficult to remember these values as you sit down at a table at home or in a restaurant. Should you be one of those who experience this problem, I suggest that you start by fixing this basic principle in your mind: *avoid white foods.*

You may think white foods are good for you because, for centuries past, the color white has been a symbol of purity. Regrettably, in the area of foods, this "purity" may mean — lacking in elements your body needs.

Science has proved, time and time again, that white processed foods are lacking in real nutritional values. And nutritionally deficient foods actually speed up the process of aging to fantastic proportions! In truth, white foods work strongly against the nine magic secrets of long life, which you are about to learn. White foods may be pleasant to taste, but they exact a terrible price in your health.

Once you have absorbed the truths about white foods which I will reveal to you in the following pages, you will be on your way to a long, healthful life. You will no longer eat badly-planned meals. You will no longer let false energy drive your physical body past the point of no return. Once again you should find yourself free of physical discomfort — able and willing to live your life to the full. Within this frame of reference, you will truly be able to say you have achieved *magic.*

A QUICK, EASY RULE

Play it safe — if it's white, don't eat it! This statement may strike a lot of my readers as rank heresy, simply because our conditioning has caused us to associate "white" with cleanliness, goodness, and purity. I have news for you. When it comes to food, white means pure, all right — pure *junk.* White manufactured food products contain little or no food value, and they can actually cause irreparable harm in the body. White food products can force your body to use up great quantities of energy to compensate for missing nutrients — nutrients present in the naturally-energized foods you should be eating.

No matter how respectable they may seem as necessities of life, the following foods should be avoided like the plague:

WHITE HARD FAT: This substance is probably the number one killer among foods. If a fat isn't in liquid form, and won't run at room temperatures, you should eliminate it from your diet, according to all competent authorities. Instead, you should use only vegetable oils in preparing foods. Medical science seems to agree that hard fats are not only more difficult to digest, but have the unhappy tendency to coat the inner linings of your arteries with a gummy substance. This gummy substance brings on disease and afflictions which substantially shorten anyone's life span. Hard fats are found in meats such as beef, pork, and lamb, and to some extent in ducks and geese.

WHITE FLOUR: This is an inert product, with nutrients removed, used mostly for making loaves of lifeless bread, or to make sweetened and larded pies and cakes. For a long life, stick to products made from whole grains, healthy brown in color, without preservatives of any kind.

WHITE SUGAR: Another inert, lifeless product, with little or no actual food value. This devitalized food may supply a "shot" of quick energy, but this is of doubtful value. When this shot wears off, you find yourself even more tired than before. Use honey, raw sugar, or any natural sweetener instead. Results will last longer and be more beneficial.

WHITE RICE: Many Oriental peoples seem only half alive. They are unfortunate examples of what happens when any diet is predominantly polished white rice. If you must eat rice, demand the rough, brown, unpolished variety, to get full value for your money.

MILK: Condemning milk may make me seem as if I dote on pushing old ladies around, but the truth is, milk is only good for babies. Once you have grown past the weaning age, drinking milk is of very doubtful merit. People who reach the age of fourteen should completely replace milk with sturdier foods. Even the traditional use of milk for those recovering from illness is now questioned.

HOW TO PUT FIRE-POWER
IN YOUR EATING HABITS

The abyss that separates sensible eating of nourishing food from over-eating is as wide as the Grand Canyon, and just as difficult to traverse. Many people are completely accustomed to eating more than is good for them. The idea of eating to live has been replaced by *living to eat.* The only time they even think of changing their meals is when the doctor says "Eat right or else!" — and this scare usually lasts for only about ten days. Many can only leave off overeating if they go into a hospital or sanitarium and are *forced* to eat less.

It seems that you cannot have both a long life and an excess of eating. You must make your own choice — adopt new eating habits, or accept a shortened life span. Give up tasty but life-shortening foods, and learn to enjoy meals of good nutritional value. Once you have done this, you will put power into your meals that can add years to your life.

Nearly everyone has heard the old saying; "He dug his grave with his teeth." This far-fetched bit of grisly humor expresses a very real, very grim truth. If you yield to the temptatation of gluttony, the traditional "god of the belly," he will reach into every nerve and fibre of your physical body to destroy you.

When overweight people are asked to change their unwholesome habits, they try to defend themselves by saying, "I work so hard I need all the food I eat to keep up my strength." The victim often makes such a statement while he wallows in useless, harmful fat.

Instead of stuffing yourself, you should form the habit of eating only what you need, in balanced nutrition. You should eat all your meals slowly and carefully, in a relaxed manner. These simples rules will help you enormously. The concept was first clearly enunciated over half a century ago by its original proponent, Horace Fletcher. At the time, his book on the subject of nutrition hit the American public like a bombshell, with the result that within months it was a common conversation piece. But, like many another great discovery, the idea soon passed into oblivion, to be revived from time to time only as a subject for humor. The humor is questionable, the idea important.

HOW TO MAKE A BALANCED
INTAKE OF FOOD
WORK FOR YOU

Obviously, the purpose and intent of *eating* should be to sustain all bodily functions at peak performance. Your physical body can absorb just so much of the life-giving qualities of food. Each nerve, cell and muscle actually requires very little *energy* in order to operate at maximum efficiency. Any attempt on your part to *force* more strength into the channels of distribution, promptly brings on stagnation.

Fortunately, for the person interested in prolonging the

life process, there is a natural *regulator* that comes as standard
equipment with each and every man, woman and child. The
trick comes in correctly *reading* the information as it is supplied by nature. To do this effectively, according to Horace
Fletcher, comes in properly *handling* our intake of food. This
practice will be fully explained in just a moment, but first, let
us describe briefly the part that each type of food plays in bringing the body up to full operational capacity.

What you are about to learn is elementary to some persons, but most competent dieticians never cease to be amazed
at the number of men and women, especially college graduates,
who are completely unfamiliar with even the basics of nutrition. Should you be one of the select few who *know* the body
temple in which you live and move and have your being, then
you can safely skip over the next paragraph, otherwise it is urgently suggested that you read and absorb the information
about to be revealed to you.

To repeat, it is well-established that there are four general classes of food. Each of these groups is endowed with a
certain life-sustaining principle. Once again, these are described as fats or oils, fruits, vegetables, and grains, plus the
one debatable source of protein — *meat*. In the beginning,
man's diet consisted almost solely of the flesh of animals that
he could stalk and kill with his crude weapons. As time passed
and the early tribes grew in comprehension, the idea that products of the soil could also be used as food gradually took hold,
until cultivation of available varieties of fruits, grains and
vegetables became a way of life.

In those early days it was noted that *meat eaters* did not
enjoy a very long life span, even when they were able to escape
the claws of animals or the stones and arrows of their enemies.
In this connection it is well to note that the length of time lived
by each individual was not influenced so much by the fact that

he was a meat eater, as it was by the steady, unvaried intake of nothing but *protein,* the principal ingredient of animal products. The physical body *demands* other active food elements such as vitamins and minerals and these can only be found in a balanced *"varietarian"* diet; including not only meat but fats or oils, fruits, vegetables and grains as well.

WILL WE ONE DAY
BE VEGETARIANS?

It is strongly asserted by vegetarians that eventually man will grow in consciousness to the point where he will no longer require meat in his diet. This is an issue I do not feel is properly a part of this discussion, so I will let it go except to say that the facts seem to favor this point of view. For most people, meat is still needed to supply a variety of protein to the diet.

In addition to the several essential elements supplied by a variety diet, there are many important *transformers,* or enzymes, which I will describe fully in my description of the first magic secret of long life.

There are at this time a growing number of research projects aimed at unlocking the secrets of this organic substance — the *enzyme* — which originates within living cells. It is a product of nature that can cause changes in other substances without being changed in its essential characteristics. Pepsin is an example of an enzyme.

There is much evidence to support the idea that the enzyme is an important *key* in the living process, but at the moment we are only concerned with attaining a long and healthy life span. Suffice to say that a balanced, *naturally* regulated diet is the only way the physical body can produce robust, life-sustaining enzymes.

HOW ONE MAN CHANGED
HIS EATING HABITS
AND EXPERIENCED A MIRACLE

Joe S. was one of many persons who attended my lectures before the national convention of the National Health Federation. The story told by Joe is typical of literally millions of persons working under pressure. With only a thirty-minute lunch break, he would gulp his food in a mad frenzy in order to rush back to his desk. "Obviously," he admitted, "my selection was based on eye-appeal more than what was good for me."

Three years of this haphazard way of eating took its toll. When I talked to Joe he was on a forced leave of absence from his job due to a rundown condition that would not respond to treatment. The very first thing he did was to include in his daily intake of food balanced portions of meat, vegetables, carbohydrates (usually a baked potato) oils (a bread spread made of safflower oil) fruits and vegetables. And to make certain he was getting the most from his food, he made it a point to stay completely relaxed during each of his meals. Within a week he informed me he was so improved he was ready to go back to work with a completely new outlook on life. By the time we reached the end of my lecture series he was using all the guidelines I am presenting in this chapter.

In the mail today I received a note from Joe that was most rewarding to me: "I am now a new person because of following your ideas about eating. Last week I received a promotion which I had never expected. I believe I am on my way to a long and happy life."

For the past forty years, some elements of the medical profession, even including at times the dominant American Medical Association, have waged a sometimes bitter campaign against health food products. They have often ridiculed those who seek nutritionally superior foods.

to chew each mouthful of food until he couldn't help swallowing the liquid that was accumulating in his mouth. Results were little short of fantastic. Within a few days improvement in his condition was so obvious that he worked out a set of "Rules for Eating" that has made history. In less than a year he was able to successfully compete with athletes half his age. Today, "Fletcherizing" is an idiom that has become part of the language. It is described in every encyclopedia of merit. It is included in thousands-upon-thousands of references covering the subject of nutrition and yet its practices are only superficially known.

For the record, we will review briefly the rules that this intrepid venturer established for himself:

(1) Eat only when hungry.
(2) Chew every mouthful of food until it practically swallows itself.
(3) Do not swallow anything that cannot be liquified.

These rules, *in action,* proved to be such a tremendous boon for Fletcher that he succeeded in stretching his life-span for nearly forty years more, but there was an Achilles Heel in his program. Just as in nearly all *original ideas,* something is left out, so it was with the idea of complete mastication of food. However, in all fairness to the man, it must be observed that at the time he made his discovery, and using only a part of one of the secrets of good living, he was enabled to nearly double his years of life with active, enjoyable enterprises.

Should you want further confirmation of the wisdom of eating slowly, turn to the ancient Talmud of the Hebrews which states, "He who eats slowly lives long."

The one vital part of the key that Fletcher left out of his pioneering in the field of nutrition will now be imparted to you as a background to the Nine Magic Secrets. *Eat a balanced diet.* If you do not know how important a balanced diet is — ask your family doctor. *Eat sparingly of all foods.* And this includes fruits, grains, vegetables — and meats. As you grow in *con-*

sciousness you will probably leave meats out of your diet, but until you can accept this *advance* in good faith, don't push your luck by "going vegetarian."

Your life span, your earning power, your sex life, even your disposition is definitely related to what you eat. Good food can provide us with powerful building blocks.

Nearly every *conscious* person is aware of the need and purpose of good food. However, an amazingly large number of men and women do not know why various edibles are important to the process of nourishing and regenerating the physical body. The mere fact that certain fruits, grains, vegetables and proteins are palatable seems to be reason enough for three or more daily sessions "at table."

To try and explain the process of "eating to live" from the beginnings of mastication, on through digestion, absorption and utilization, would require a lengthy comment, most of which is far too technical for most persons to understand, much less interpret intelligently. Why not "zero in" on the most important factor of nutrition — the end result — in relation to the attainment of a long, active, and enjoyable period of confident living?

Most competent doctors are now willing to admit that good food does really determine how we live our lives, how we act or react when we are dealing with others, and even how successful we will be in our business or professional activities and most important "how long we will live."

YOUR SOURCES OF
VIBRANT ENERGY

Again, it might seem to be an over-simplification, but there are only four general classes of good foods which are essential building blocks in creating a long and enjoyable life. They are: (1) Fats or oils (2) Starches or carbohydrates (3) Fruits and vegetables (4) Proteins.

Two psychiatrists associated with the National Institute of Health at Bethesda, Maryland, stress the fact that food preferences reveal a person's capacity for earning power and leadership as well as his ability to get along with his associates. Some hardnosed American businessmen expect that before too long *food preference* of an applicant will be included along with aptitude and intelligence tests, as a part of his *qualification examination.*

Bob H. told me he tried out the idea in his factory, employing two hundred persons, with startling results. According to Bob's report, absenteeism was reduced 30% during the first year; grieviences tapered off to almost nothing; personality clashes lessened to the point where they were the exception instead of the rule — and the greatest benefit of all: production increased a sturdy 12% above previous years.

Food preferences as keys to a person's behavior are still somewhat general, but for the most part it is known that:

(1) Vegetarians usually avoid social situations, are ordinarily quite reserved, and, for the most part, avoid competitive drive.

(2) Persons who prefer green vegetables such as Romaine lettuce, spinach, string beans and zucchini are normally more reasonable than others.

(3) Persons who lean toward meats or other high protein foods tend to be more aggressive, enthusiastic, and action oriented. Leadership qualities are also more in evidence in this group.

(4) Persons who favor mixed vegetable dishes such as corn, lima beans and string beans are usually more likely to be involved in office romances.

MY DISCOVERIES ABOUT FOOD

Let me summarize my discoveries about the role of food in good health:

(1) Food is essential to the living process. Because the body chemistry of each person is different, the kind and variety of food you eat must be your own decision.

(2) For good health and long life, everyone's body requires a balanced intake of fats, carbohydrates, fruits, vegetables and proteins.

(3) Although there is a wide diversity of views and theories advanced in support of processed foods, the truth is that *the nearer any given food item is to its natural state, the better nutritional values it offers the consumer.*

(4) For the purpose of conserving body energies and prolonging life, every mouthful of food should be chewed until it practically swallows itself.

(5) As you become conscious of the merits of sensible eating habits, and begin to follow these suggestions in practice, you will before long begin to eat only what you need, when you are truly hungry.

(6) When you follow these rules, you are fully prepared to get the most out of the Nine Magic Health Secrets which I am about to reveal.

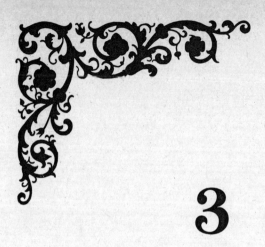

3

THE FIRST
MAGIC HEALTH SECRET:
REJUVENATING POWER OF
FIVE TROPICAL FRUITS

Every tropical fruit known to man has at least one magic life-sustaining property. This special ingredient can run the whole scale of vitamins, minerals, and enzymes. Which product of nature is best for you can only be determined by extensive testing supervised by your doctor, or by your own personal reaction.

HOW TO FIND THE
REAL FOUNTAIN OF YOUTH

Fortunately for all of us, the bounty of nature does provide for our use a magic array of life-giving foods. For example, the *real fountain of youth* is in the juices or body of five well-known fruits. These are papaya, bread fruit, pineapple, bananas, and mangoes. All of them are often found in the fruit and vegetable section of a well-stocked grocery store. The choice of which one to eat is yours. My favorite is the *papaya* because of its high concentration of enzymes helpful in the process of digestion.

For a thousand generations, the papaya, this magical melon, a native of the tropics, has been used for its health-sustaining powers. All over the world men and women conscious of the need for enzymes are now recognizing this versatile fruit not only as a digestive aid, but also because it possesses a wide range of health benefits unknown until the papaya research project of Chester D. French.[1]

It is claimed by researchers, including French, that the papaya melon not only possesses preventive qualities, because of its vitamin-mineral content, but it also tends to stimulate all of the other body processes into more efficient activity.

Serious researchers who have delved into the merits of the papaya melon have proved that this unusual fruit contains all of the vitamins in healthful quantities plus an excellent source of natural protein.

When we begin to review the list of benefits that can be achieved simply by eating the melon or drinking the juice of the fruit, I will begin with the story of John M. who signed up for my class in Better Living, but, for reasons unknown to me at the time, was not too regular in his attendance. Quite by accident, John chanced to show up the day I lectured on *enzymes*. In my discussion, I pointed out that the papaya melon was high in digestive enzymes. At the time, John made no comment, but I learned later that he found a dehydrated form of the papaya enzyme in the local health food store. By follow-

---

[1]Chester D. French, chief researcher for Frenco, Inc., Dallas, Texas (a manufacturer of more than 100 products derived from the papaya melon).

ing directions carefully, he managed to solve his problem. It seems he had suffered from constipation for years with the situation getting so bad at times that he would get groggy to the point of actually becoming ill, too ill, in fact, to either work or attend classes. Within a week he informed me he began to feel like a new man. He went on to explain that he no longer had to take harsh laxatives. The enzyme tablets were doing so well for him that his general health was improving by the day. "You can bet I won't miss another lecture," he declared and with that he stepped briskly from the classroom at the end of that session.

In addition to the forgoing, the papaya melon also has the reputation for eliminating chronic dyspepsia. It relieves the immediate problem and gradually improves and returns the digestive system to normal.

D.R. writes me from Oregon that "for years I was troubled with a *sour* stomach after my luncheon or evening meal. So much, in fact, that I had to keep a supply of anti-acid tablets on hand at all times. Without them I was in misery. When I learned about the 'magic melon' from one of your radio broadcasts, I sought out the largest health food store in Portland where I obtained a bottle of enzyme tablets. Taking them according to directions on the label, I began to notice an immediate improvement. Within a week, all of my problems of digestion had disappeared completely. For once, I was glad I took the time to listen to a radio program."

The papaya melon thrives profusely in parts of the Hawaiian Islands, usually in great clusters.

The word, "enzyme" comes from the Greek *enzymos,* which means among other things, to agitate. The process of *stirring up* is to cause a change. Within our present frame of reference, it means to stimulate digestion.

The vast army of enzymes your body produces acts as a guardian of the gate — your mouth. With your first bite of food, your precious salivary glands begin to deliver the potent digestive aids we call enzymes. This is the first step toward properly digesting the food you eat. Should you require a good reason for chewing each mouthful of food until it practically swallows itself — *this is it.* Failure to meet this first requisite of eating to live means that enzymes in your saliva won't have time to work and your intake of nourishment will not be properly digested. In other words, you avoid digestive upsets by slow eating.

Probably the biggest argument against processed foods derives from the fact that all of the natural enzymes are destroyed in the preparation of the edible materials for marketing. *Enzymes are your key to long life,* so choosing foods for enzymes is vital.

It is also important to be active, because enzymes must be spurred into peak performance if they are to fulfill their real purpose. This can be easily accomplished by body movement. Walking, stretching, doing tensing exercises or performing ordinary duties, *other than sitting,* will do the job. When enzymes are not stimulated into action, they have a tendency to become simply nonreacting compounds, organic in nature. The end result is that they contribute nothing to your bodily functions. If you wonder why anyone should exercise, even moderately, you now have a logical answer.

Every edible fruit and vegetable is known to produce one or more valuable enzymes. The enzyme, *peroxidase* increases life expectancy to a very marked degree. This tremendously potent enzyme is present in the Fuerte avocado in very large amounts, especially when the avocado is ripe. Other vegetables rich in this essential enzyme are freshly picked green peas, cauliflower, tomatoes, asparagus, and alfalfa sprouts.

In the metabolic process, peroxidase is potent because it acts as a catalyst in holding down concentrations of peroxide. Peroxide in your system should be kept at safe levels — levels that are not damaging to brain cells. Damaged brain cells are the chief cause of mental deterioration.

In addition to the enzymes provided by nature, each organ of your body contributes a valuable enzyme. With each bite of food you swallow, an enzyme is changed into a new form. When a particular vitamin or mineral is isolated from the food you eat, it is transferred to the body unit in need of the energy it supplies.

The five tropical fruits, papayas, bread fruits, pineapples, bananas, and mangoes, have rejuvenating power because of the enzymes they contain.

THE ROYAL FAMILY OF ENZYMES

It is generally agreed that the human body is host to well over 700 enzymes — each with a different function to perform. All these enzymes, working together, sustain the living process. When you eat, enzymes begin to work on the foods you supply and promptly transform the proteins, vegetables, carbohydrates and fruits into life-prolonging substances. Glandular action in your body would soon cease without the help of enzymes.

You have within you an enzyme that helps to build phosphorus, a mineral, into your bone and nerve material. Another enzyme aids in fixing *iron* in your blood cells. If you suffer from a low blood count or conditions of anemia, you should know that not only must you include food supplements rich in iron at every meal, but you must have an active enzymatic system. This is needed in order to metabolize the iron you take for use in the blood stream.

HOW TO BUILD ENZYME POWER

Where does your body find the materials from which the enzymes are created? There are only three sources: the food you eat — the water you drink — and the air you breathe.

Obviously, there are certain substances in air and water and food which aid in the formation of enzymes. Raw foods are a rich source of effective enzymes.

Unfortunately, foods lose some of the essential enzymes when they are cooked. Heat destroys enzymes at an alarming rate under certain conditions. Therefore, it should be clear that the less heat you use in the preparation of fruits and vegetables the better off you will be.

The first magic health secret is to maintain your enzyme level by eating lots of fruits and vegetables with a minimum of cooking.

Many medical and research authorities believe that most diseases begin when enzymes are lost or are deficient in strength. "In addition to the digestive enzymes," Harry W. Edgerton, M.D., declares, "you must have a balanced array of enzymes waiting in other cells. This means catalysts that take over after the foods you eat have all been changed into usable form by your body cells. These catalysts continue the job of changing the digested food into materials the body needs in order to continue in good working order."

In other words, there are important enzymes in your body. You must eat foods that keep bringing valuable enzymes into your system for long life and good health.

WHY ENZYMES ARE IMPORTANT
TO YOUR LONG LIFE

When your "mouth waters" it means a very valuable enzyme is flowing. It is called *saliva*. This number one digestive generator contains the enzyme we know as *ptyalin*. This is the first step in the digestive process. Carbohydrates or starches are set upon by ptyalin in order to break them down to a more usable form called maltose. Should you bolt your food without proper chewing, then *ptyalin* is unable to perform its rightful function. When this happens, unchewed foods high in starch content will reach your stomach poorly prepared for its acid content. In fact, the stomach enzyme may counteract whatever *ptyalin* was supposed to accomplish. This can bring on stomach pains, induce a feeling of heaviness and a completely listless feeling after your meal.

The one enzyme which stands tall in the entire system of protein digestion is *pepsin*. This divides the proteins into two types known as *proteoses* and *peptones*.

The enzyme known as lipase is number three in the scheme of digestion. *Lipase* serves the purpose of splitting fats or oils. They become a valuable aid to skin tone. In new form, they serve to nourish skin cells, cushion the effects of bruises, ward off infectious virus cells and help allergic conditions.

Another equally valuable member of the enzyme family is released by the pancreas, so it is called *pancreatic lipase*. This essential enzyme acts upon fats that have already been emulsified by bile and transforms them into fatty acids and *glycerol*. Pancreatic lipase is the only effective fat-splitting enzyme.

The pancreas also produces *trypsin*. The job of trypsin is to act on foods which have only been partially digested in the stomach. Trypsin also helps digest food which are short in the enzyme pepsin.

Rennin is another important member of the enzyme family. Its job is to cause the coagulation of milk. This action changes its protein into casein, a form that is usable by your body.

Another pancreatic enzyme is *amylase*. Its purpose is to split uncooked starch or carbohydrates into maltose. Its function is important to good digestion.

All enzymes are named according to the food substance that they must digest. Accordingly, sucrase is an enzyme that breaks down sugar into a form the body can use. The enzyme *sucrase* brings on a change in the presence of phosphorus which is called *phosphatase.*

A very special intestinal enzyme known as *invertase* has the ability to break down a million times its own weight in sugar and be ready and waiting for more.[2]

Hydrochloric acid is a substance in the stomach. Most persons do not think of *hydrochloric acid* as an enzyme, but it is one of the most valuable. The secretion of this enzyme is related to the acid base balance of the body, consequently it is linked to the elimination of an acid urine by the kidneys. Good breathing tends to eliminate alkaline gas. The big job of hydrochloric acid is to work primarily upon tough foods. This includes such foods as fibrous meats, vegetables and poultries. When you are short of this valuable stomach enzyme, you run the grave risk of improperly digesting your food and losing the vitamins and proteins which your body must have in order to sustain good health. It is known that persons who are fond of tomatoes, *without sugar,* rarely find themselves lacking hydrochloric acid.

Procollagenase is another enzyme that has been isolated and is being used to eliminate disfiguring scars and remove intestinal adhesions after surgery. Your doctor can inform you on how best to use this valuable enzyme.

It is now claimed that the enzyme *fibrinolysin* will dissolve leg blood clots. This depends upon how soon after formation of the clot the enzyme is used. It is also believed that this same enzyme can be administered in order to dissolve coronary clots or clogged cerebral arteries that tend to bring on heart attacks or strokes. Valuable research is making great progress in this field.

Bromelin, an enzyme found in pineapple stems, has been helpful to women who suffer menstrual pains.

---

[2]Harry W. Edgerton, M.D., asserts that too many "high" colonics wash away this valuable enzyme.

Such conditions as hemorrhoids, heart disease, skin allergies and bed sores have been treated with *papain*. The enzyme is taken from the ordinary papaya melon. Papain helps to reduce inflamed hemorrhoids by dissolving fibrin deposits. This serves to drain the fluids that caused the swelling so that the useless dead cells can be removed. It is now claimed that the enzyme papain, because of its dissolving power, may even overcome the condition of a slipped disc by dissolving the misplaced disc substance.

Fibrinolysin, the blood enzyme, as I stated before, serves to break up certain fibrinous growths as well as clots. From this same source the enzyme *ribonuclease* is used to help do away with such fibrous elements. This product derives from beef pancreas and is available in drug stores under the trade name of *Dorhase.* A prescription from your doctor is required.

The one outstanding enzyme in the royal family of enzymes is *peroxidase.* The chief claim to .fame of this health guardian lies in the fact that it slows down mental deterioration in a most remarkable manner. I have only actually witnessed two rather startling instances wherein amazing recoveries were in evidence. Carl L. and Don W. were members of my class group in the Institute of Lifetime Learning. Both men were in their early eighties and they appeared to be slipping fast in mental abilities. Both men limped badly and had to use canes for support. When I gave my lecture on the value of enzymes in raw or lightly cooked foods, they were unusually attentive. Because most of the persons who signed up for my classes were well along in years, I stressed the need for the enzyme peroxidase. As I have previously explained, this potent enzyme is known to be present in important amounts in avocados, cauliflower, fresh garden peas, and alfalfa sprouts. I suggested that Don and Carl include all four items in their daily intake of food. Both men promptly followed this advice. Within a week the improvement in these two men was so obvious that it created quite a sensation among my class members.

Today Don is as mentally alert and perceptive as a man half his age, and Carl has signed up for a class in Political Science where the entrance requirements are rather stiff.

Jane W. of Iowa tells me that her mother, age 82, was rapidly approaching a condition described as "senile." Jane had, by chance, caught my broadcast in which I explained that I always include in my salads a tablespoon or two of raw peas, a tablespoon or two of grated cauliflower, and at least a quarter of a ripe avocado. "The idea sounded 'way-out'" she admits. "But anything was worth a try. Getting mother to add raw vegetables to her diet of meat and potatoes was quite a chore, but gradually she accepted the new foods."

Jane's mother was gently "forced" to try her daughter's suggestions, largely because she wasn't served her favorite dishes until she had eaten her salad. "Improvement wasn't too noticeable at first," Jane went on, "but within a month mother began to show evidence of becoming her old active and alert self. A year has now passed and she is taking part in church functions and family social events."

All enzymes have magic properties. Enzymes are said to have produced remarkable results with Parkinson's disease when something goes wrong with the nerve ganglia at the base of the brain. Evidence seems to indicate that the brains of persons stricken with this disease manifested unusually low concentrations of two closely related chemicals identified as *dopamine* and *serotonin*. For purposes of research it was assumed that a deficiency of an enzyme called dopa-decarboxylase might be responsible. However, remarkable recoveries have been reported when this enzyme in combination with others have been used under proper medical supervision.

Two other *valuable pancreatic enzymes,* known to your doctor as *trypsin* and *chymotrypsin,* are used to offset inflammation and reduce swelling. A major packing company has developed *chrymotrysin* in a special form. The purpose of the new product is to be used during cataract surgery. In this delicate operation, the surgeon must remove the diseased lens. When he uses this enzyme there is a chance he may not have to cut the tiny ligaments that hold the lens in place. Instead, the surgeon can inject chrymotrypsin. This enzyme helper then selectively dissolves the anchor fibers, so that the lens can float loose and be removed.

Hepatitis, an infectious disease that attacks the liver, brings on an abnormal increase in the enzyme *glutamic pyruvic transaminase*. The growth in the blood stream can be as much as ten times normal. When the attending physician takes blood tests at various intervals following his first diagnosis, he can actually determine the rate at which the disease is developing. This information guides him in prescribing treatment. This is accomplished by following the enzyme count.

It is now theorized that *histidase* also acts as a bulwark against retardation. A deficiency of this enzyme histidase has an influence upon the ability to learn or remember. Source of this wonder product of nature can be found in fresh fruits, especially apples.

Another example of an important enzyme is known as *thyroxin*. It is a basic product of the thyroid glands.

A common mental disturbance known as *schizophrenia*, is responding favorably to enzyme treatment. The affliction is apparently brought on by a deficiency of the enzyme *cholinesterase*.

It is now accepted by many doctors, perhaps hopefully, that by simple injection or administration of this enzyme by a competent doctor, a patient could be cured.

HOW YOU CAN
PROTECT YOURSELF
AGAINST DISEASE

Under your doctor's supervision you can begin to increase your intake of the enzyme *catalase*. This potent enzyme, as well

as most others, is destroyed by heat. *Garlic is rich in catalase.*
Eating garlic frequently is good for you — if you can use it
freely without destroying your social standing. Luckily, it is
also available in tablets which cause no odor. It is almost axio-
matic that the sedentary person is one with a low supply of
catalase. A brisk twenty-block walk is one way of increasing
your oxygen consumption. In this manner you can provide an
environment favorable to catalase. Your body cells and tissues
require oxygen in order to form and manufacture this essential
enzyme.

The polluted air we breathe, the habit of smoking we indulge, or the processed foods we eat, interfere with our cata-
lase-peroxide balance. It is not only the catalase enzyme which
is destroyed, but the nutritional values of the food we eat. Start
now to reduce your intake of these substances, which slow down
or destroy the beneficial action of this valuable enzyme.

THE INNER GUARDIANS
OF LONG LIFE

It should now be clear that enzymes sustain just about
every body function. We need them to maintain life and health.
Enzymes take the food we eat and transform it into muscle,
nerve and bone. Glandular action would cease without these
natural aids to good health.

For example, each of us has an enzyme that helps to build
phosphorus, a mineral, into bone and nerve material. Another
enzyme aids in fixing iron in your blood cells. Those who suffer
from a low blood count or conditions of anemia should know
that not only must food supplements rich in iron be eaten at
every meal but it is also equally necessary to have an active
enzymatic system.

THE DISEASE FIGHTING
POWERS OF ENZYMES

An excellent example of this fact is revealed in your digestive system. Insulin is required to dissolve and metabolize sugars. Without insulin, too much sugar enters into the blood stream. When this happens you may even suffer a coma. And this is only one of a multitude of unpleasant situations produced by insulin shortage. Obviously, you need the full cooperation of every enzyme in your body in order to carry on the life processes.

When disease enters the body it happens because of the quality of or lack of the enzymes your body has created. Enzymes play a powerful role in warding off disease. You can help them do a good job. Nearly all enzymes that have been isolated are *lytic*. This means that they dissolve some type of food into molecules that can be used by the body for proper functioning.

In reviewing the list of benefits that can be achieved simply by eating the pulp or drinking the juices of the five magical fruits of the tropics, you will find the bounty of nature is unlimited.

BEGIN NOW TO PUT THE POWERFUL ARMY OF ENZYMES TO WORK FOR YOU.

THOUGHTS ABOUT
THE FIRST MAGIC SECRET

(1) Tropical fruits such as breadfruit, pineapple, bananas, mangoes and papayas are valuable sources of *enzymes*. Your health and long life depend upon enzymes.

(2) There are three sources of enzyme power — water, air and healthful foods.

(3) Certain substances in air, water and food can aid your body in the formation of enzymes. Certain raw foods are a rich source of enzymes. Papaya, for example, provides digestive enzymes.

(4) Digestive enzymes, such as are found in fruits such as papayas, influence your taste buds favorably.

(5) Your thoughts at mealtime should be happy, since negative emotions will slow down the secretion of enzymes.

(6) Enzymes affect the products of your body's glandular system. Without question, the enzymes produced by eating raw tropical fruit increase your chances for a long, happy life.

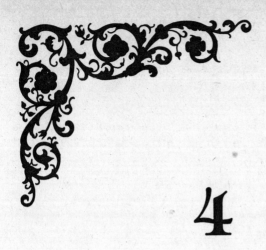

4

THE SECOND
MAGIC HEALTH SECRET:
MYSTERY OF THE GREEN LIGHT

My introduction to the magic of the green light came about in a most dramatic manner.

Several years ago I was suffering from a severe internal infection in my heel. Shots and painkillers failed to offer any relief. One day a friend told me about the *green magic,* known as chlorophyll. When I questioned my doctor about chlorophyll being used in this way, he had to admit that he had never heard of the product being taken for this purpose. However, acute pain made me willing to try anything. On a quick trip to my local health food store, I found the green concentrate readily available in liquid form. I followed directions carefully as stated on the label and within a few days all pain was gone. Apparently the infection was healed, because I have not been troubled since.

Naturally enough, the question now will be: Can chlorophyll be taken safely when any internal infection is present? Obviously, the first thing you should do is see your doctor, but from all the evidence studied so far it won't do any harm should you begin taking this "green magic health secret" at once.

Unfortunately, most of the research directed toward this valuable product of nature is so recent that only a small number of the nation's medical doctors have ever heard of the green juice extracted from plants being used as a healer. However, so much evidence has been gathered within recent months supporting the medicinal value of chlorophyll that its use is spreading rapidly.

One lady in Arizona reports that her father developed a running sore on the side of his face about the size of a quarter that refused to heal. In one of my TV talk shows I mentioned the growing interest in the apparently magic qualities of chlorophyll both for internal and external use. When Mrs. M. heard my comments about this amazing product of nature, she promptly sought out a health food store and purchased a bottle of the liquid sunshine. Later, she informed me that she followed directions on the label quite generously, but she also daubed the solution full-strength on the reluctant lesion with startling results. Within a matter of a very few days the troublesome sore healed over — "and" she declared happily, "it has never returned."

RIDDLE OF THE AGES SOLVED

For ages we have wondered where all of the beautiful green color in nature comes from. To solve this problem an

enterprising chemist began a series of tests. Before long he was
able to segregate the green coloring in leaves and grasses. He
took the Greek word *chloros,* meaning green, and a second
Greek work *phyll,* meaning leaf, and called his discovery
chlorophyll. A new word was born and a miracle product of
nature was created for our use.

World famous executive, Charles F. Kettering, once went
on record to declare, "If we knew how chlorophyll, the green
pigment in plants, is able to transform sunlight, water, and
carbon dioxide into food sugars, we could transform civiliza-
tion overnight."

Many distinguished scientists and serious researchers
have witnessed this second magic health secret — the healing
powers of chlorophyll. Deep-lying infections have responded
favorably to the green magic within days. Open wounds have
been cleansed of all septicity within hours. Chronic sinus conditions have been relieved within a few weeks. Inflamation of
the mucus membrane, seat of the common cold, has been reduced dramatically within hours. And ordinary skin infections
have responded to applications of chlorophyll in a matter of
minutes with no irritating or toxic after effects.

Strangely enough, chlorophyll is comparatively new in
the healing arts. Although it is known that this basic color of
nature is as old as life on our planet, until recently little has
been known of its therapeutic qualities.

To the ordinary person, the idea of using the green juice
of plants for healing purposes is like something out of a book
of magic. During the past century many doctors and distin-
gusihed men of science have reported literally hundreds of
cases where deep-lying infections have responded favorably to
some combination of chlorophyll. It has been used to cleanse
open wounds. It has been used in atomizers for the relief of
sinus trouble. It has greatly reduced inflammation of the mucus
membrane in persons afflicted with common head colds. And

even more amazing is the rapid and effective healing that is accomplished.

One day Roger B. phoned me from Iowa to tell me about his experience with chlorophyll. "For several years," he disclosed to me, "I suffered from painful running sores on my left leg. When I learned about the 'green juice' experiments from you in one of your talks before the National Health Federation, I decided to give the product a try. It took some searching, but I finally located a firm in Anaheim, California, able to supply me with two pints of the so-called 'magic.'" Roger admitted he was somewhat dubious at first, especially when a week passed with no apparent change. Then, all-of-a-sudden the sores stopped oozing and the twice-a-day change of bandages was no longer necessary. At the end of four weeks nothing remained but dried scabs. "Nearly a year has passed now and the problem has not returned to plague me." Roger reports. "I am eternally grateful."

THE SOURCE OF
GROWTH AND LIFE

At the present time we do know that when the sunlight comes to earth, all plant life begins to grow. Instantly the miracle of life is created because the green magic of chlorophyll is revealed. Within the emerging plant, strange things begin to happen. Water and carbon dioxide gas are separated — a feat which skilled chemists find difficult and expensive. Truly, it is a miracle of nature.

With the foregoing hypothesis in mind the noted German scientist, Dr. Richard Willstatter, reasoned that since all life energy comes from the sun, the next logical step could be to solve the secret of plant growth. "How," he wanted to know," is the magic in which solar energy is captured and passed on to all living things accomplished?" The happy result of his probings revealed the substance we know as chlorophyll.

When you come to think about it, the law of creation takes over, with only a lifeless gas and water to work with! These two elements are transformed, as if by magic, into useful energy. Within this basic combination all manner of miracles are wrought. Fresh oxygen is released from plants. Trees and grasses revitalize our polluted air. Units of energy that we know as vitamins, minerals, and carbohydrates are formed. All of these natural benefits are rapidly created and stored up in the living plant.

A NATURAL ANTISEPTIC

Most commercial antiseptics are counter irritants. On the other hand, chlorophyll is at once strong and yet mild. When applied in full strength to wounded body tissues, it tends to exterminate the germs and bacteria that breed disease without burning tissues. Common antiseptics merely irritate body tissues and create new problems. With an ever-ready bottle of green magic handy to be used as a gargle, a spray, or gently swabbed on injured or inflamed tissues, the results are little short of a miracle. Precisely how nature accomplishes her magic is still her guarded secret.

How safe is chlorophyll to use when you "catch" a common cold? Should you wish to be absolutely safe, have your doctor check your problem — especially when your situation is anything more than an ordinary flu bug or head cold. If you are told yours is "just a cold," ask about using chlorophyll to treat it. You are entitled to a reasonable answer.

Ginger B., one of my class members, reported her experience with chlorophyll. One morning when she awakened she found herself on the verge of a very heavy cold. She remember-ed hearing another member of the group tell of her *"swab-and-gargle"* stunt and decided to try it. Ginger took an ordinary cotton swab obtainable in any drug store, dipped the tip in chlorophyll and swabbed out her nasal passages as far back as she could reach without injury. During that day, Ginger re-peated this process several times. In the meantime she gargled with pure chlorophyll about every hour. When she awakened the next morning all symptoms of her cold had disappeared. Since that time she has been a strong booster for the healing powers of the *green magic.*

How safe is chlorophyll to use as a douche in matters of feminine hygiene?

Reports from all clinical testing I could find, stated that many unpleasant feminine hygiene conditions responded favorably to this form of cleansing treatment when a strong solution of the green magic was used.

A lady brought this question up during a class discussion. A few of the women present maintained that the green magic was nothing more than a contraceptive, while others were equally emphatic in declaring chlorophyll was the most power-ful cleanser and deodorant they had ever used. Today whether or not the green magic is a contraceptive is no longer debat-able. *It is not!* Instead, "it really helps — not only as a deodor-ant in matters of cleanliness, but it also helps to neutralize any possible toxic materials that might interfere with developing a perfectly normal baby."

In my class groups the question was often asked, "Is chlorophyll safe to use as a mouth-wash or gargle?"

Many authorities claim trench mouth or pyorrhea will respond favorably to a full strength solution of the green magic. I know that since I have been rinsing my mouth at least once each day I have had no oral problems. All evidence at this time indicates that improvement can be noted within one or two days. However, when you have had a tooth pulled or oral surgery performed, it is best to follow the advice of your dentist.

Joan W. returned from a camping trip with the inside of her mouth so raw it was painful to eat. A fast trip to her family doctor who, fortunately, happened to be an especially knowledgable practitioner, suggested that she try gargling with an undiluted solution of chlorophyll. "Within hours," she reported, "the irritation began to lessen and next morning all of the inflamation was gone."

In class one day, James O. raised the question, "How safe is chlorophyll to use when a person is known to have peptic or gastric ulcer?" He was growing tired of a "milk diet."

At that time, I really had no pat answer, but have learned since that many doctors report rapid healing when a tablespoonful of liquid chlorophyll is taken in about four ounces of warm water every two or three hours.

Since James had been having a very rough time with an extremely painful and disturbing ulcer, he decided to give the green magic a try — especially when he was assured that no toxic or side effects had ever been reported. When class convened the following week, James was a very happy person. "I'm feeling better by the day," he declared. "I'm now able to eat something besides soft foods, and if I never drink another glass of milk, that will be soon enough!"

Another often-asked question invariably comes up: "Will chlorophyll be helpful in treating my arthritis?"

Since this is a question that is open to considerable debate, all I can do is relate to you the facts as I know them. At this time it is indicated that sufferers take a tablespoonful of chlorophyll mixed with a small glass of water before each meal. They often experience remarkable relief.

I recall one instance when a member of our group, whom we shall call Linda G., admitted that she had been in con-

siderable pain during most of her waking hours until she heard
about the green magic. "Within a week," she stated quite simply, "my arthritis began to disappear. I no longer had to take
aspirin for even temporary relief — and today I feel like a
million!"

All too often the question is asked, "Will chlorophyll in-
jure healthy tissue?"

From all the information I can gather, the sum total of
the experiments conducted so far, it has been established re-
peatedly that there were absolutely no toxic or side effects of
any kind in evidence. Chlorophyll is known to be gentle to
body tissues.

Since chlorophyll is so closely related to hemoglobin,
according to competent authorities, it has been proved in most
instances that the red blood count will return to normal with
the administration of heavy doses of chlorophyll. In fact, in
every instance where controlled testing was applied, the red
cell count returned to normal within four to five days, even
when an anemic condition was known to exist.

"GREEN MAGIC"
AS A DEODORANT

It is now fairly well established that chlorophyll is both
a breath and body sweetener. When the green magic is used
generously, unpleasant body odors are reduced almost to a
minimum. During one of our class discussion periods, Jane O.
volunteered the information that for years she had suffered
from a most vexing odor problem. In fact she was frank to admit that it interfered with her social activities, her sex life, even
her physical comfort. "I tried every deodorant on the market,
special soaps supposed to lessen body odors, but nothing

seemed to solve the problem. Then one day a friend told me about chlorophyll. Within a very few days after starting to put a tablespoon of the green magic in a small glass of water several times each day and drinking it, life began to change for me. Friends no longer avoided me and tonight I am stepping out with a brand-new boyfriend. Actually, I am living once again — and all because of this wonderful natural product of nature."

THE ELIXIR OF YOUTH
DISCOVERED

During the centuries all manner of brews, tonics and stimulants of doubtful value have been foisted upon the public. Some of these mixtures were herbal compounds capable of accomplishing some good, but for the most part, the so-called tonics were without merit. Most of the claimed powers of the blends were figments of the makers' imagination. In early America the traveling medicine man was commonplace in rural communities. These practitioners of guile did not know that the fields of new mown hay passed in their travels contained a gold mine of healing elements. Most of us know that when an animal is sick, it will eat grass. There has to be a reason. Perhaps some of you will remember the story of King Nebuchadnezzer. Plagued with illness, he was advised to go into the fields to live on grass. Apparently the ancients had knowledge of the healing power of the *green magic*.

An eminent research scientist associated with Ketterling has described chlorophyll as "concentrated sun power." In fact, he goes on to assert, "Chlorophyll increases and sustains the functions of the heart, favorably affects the workings of the intestines, and helps to cleanse the uterus and lungs. "This, he declares, "is accomplished by raising the basic nitrogen exchange, and is therefore a tonic of great value."

When you consider all of the other qualities of chlorophyll, including its stimulating properties, it can truly be classed as one of the magic products of nature.

YOUR GREEN KEY
TO GOOD HEALTH

It is generally an accepted fact that anaerobic bacteria, disease-producing micro-organisms that somehow manage to survive in all-too-many human bodies, cannot exist in the presence of oxygen, or oxygen-producing agents. Chlorophyll is just such a natural magic oxygen-producing substance.

One researcher declared, "Bacteria being of vegetable origin, yet possessing no chlorophyll ordinarily, *undergo some biological change in the presence of this substance.*" According to this conclusion, we believe it is safe to assume that some valid effect is produced when chlorophyll comes in contact with body tissues, regardless of whether those tissues are normal or infected. Chlorophyll appears to exercise a normalizing influence on all body tissues.

With all the magic powers of chlorophyll, it appears that the product is completely nontoxic, and very definitely devoid of all unpleasant side effects.

THE MAGIC INGREDIENT
OF A COMMON FIELD CROP

One of the profound secrets of nature is the kinship between sunlight and the green plants of the earth. When this kinship is better understood, science believes man will be brought closer to conquering all manner of infections.

The common field crop, alfalfa, is an excellent source of chlorophyll. All that the growing alfalfa has to do to bring you this rich, life-giving fluid is to absorb sunlight, take in water and minerals from the soil through its root system, and presto! — we have the amazing substance, chlorophyll.

Alfalfa that is grown in richly composted soil, without the use of chemical sprays or artificial fertilizers, yields a near perfect form of chlorophyll. When you buy freshly-pressed juice, bottled without any preservatives, you are getting the best possible product.

THOUGHTS ABOUT
THE SECOND MAGIC SECRET

(1) The magic of concentrated sun power is in chlorophyll, found in green plants. Chlorophyll seems to have remarkable powers in clearing up infections.

(2) Chlorophyll in liquid form is easily obtained and can be used internally and externally.

(3) This plant-derived substance speeds healing of wounds, reduces inflammation, and cleans the skin. It seems to be a natural antiseptic, and is a very effective deodorant.

(4) Chlorophyll seems helpful in relieving arthritis.

(5) This substance can be considered a real *elixer of youth* in the way it fights off infection and stimulates the production of red cells.

5

THE THIRD
MAGIC HEALTH SECRET:
THE GREAT EMULSIFIER

A REMARKABLE DISCOVERY OF
HEALTH AND FOOD VALUES

In searching the musty records of history, we find that the ancient Chinese were the first to know of the unusual food qualities of soybeans. For thousands of years these so-called "backward people" have used soybeans, not only for dependable nourishment, but also to make a tasty form of "milk" for baby feeding.

The most dramatic claims for this "magic" health secret involves its use as a source of lecithin. However, there are other valuable nutrients in soybeans. In fact, this lowly legume is a complete source of food in its own right.

Competent research in this area has revealed some rather unusual food qualities. For example, the protein content of soybeans is eleven times greater than milk — nearly twice as much as lima or navy beans — and three times greater than eggs.

Soybean oil is highly desirable in cooking, salad-making, and baking. The dry soybean contains from 15% to 20% usable oil. It is important in the ordinary diet because it contains certain vitamins such as A and D. It is also an excellent source of physical energy. In addition to this characteristic, it is a good source of the valuable E vitamin.

According to N.A. Ferri, M.D., foremost among the phospholipids are lecithin and cephalin which are especially abundant in the brain, heart, muscles, kidneys, bone marrow, spinal cord and liver. The phospholipids are also present in the endocrine glands and especially the gonads. Lecithin and cephalin are essential not only for the tissue organs of the nervous and glandular systems in all living organisms, but they are regarded also as the most effective generators of great physical, mental and glandular energy.

Mrs. W., writing to me from Nebraska, informs me that when she added soybean products to the family's diet, the general health of all members was noticeably improved within a matter of weeks. "In fact," she declared, "my husband, who was slowing down perceptibly, seemed to take a new lease on life — so much so that he was able to resume his conjugal activities with zest and enthusiasm."

As a food product, the whole soybean is rich in vitamins and minerals. This includes calcium, phosphorus, and natural iron. This quality remains stable even when the bean is ground into soy flour, or processed into grits. The green soybeans are known to contain vitamins A, B, and a small quantity of C. Unfortunately, the dry bean loses its C content, but makes up for this deficiency with about three times as much of the essential B vitamin.

HOW EMULSIFYING HELPS LONGER LIFE

Today great numbers of health-minded persons have discovered this magic health secret. When the emulsifying qualities of lecithin become better known, however, it will grow even more in popularity. A steadily increasing number of men and women interested in good health are turning to the use of soybean oil in place of the old-fashioned hard fats coming from meat and butterfat. More and more substitutes for milk, butter, cheese and other dairy-type products are being made from soybean oil.

THESE PRODUCTS ARE NATURAL FOODS, NOT IMITATIONS

Contrary to the propaganda dispensed by some self-styled authorities, foods derived from soybeans are not *imitations* or substitutes. They should not be labeled as artificial meat. They are rich in protein and fat in vegetable form in their own right. They can provide satisfactory nutrition either as a replacement for the imagined need for meat when food requirements indicate a change would be helpful, or for persons who are vegetarians.

Lecithin, a nutrient derived from cold-pressed soybeans,

is now proving to be valuable in certain corrective diets. This is apparently true because it contains valuable amounts of phosphorus, inositol, and choline. All are essential to normal body functioning. Unfortunately, biochemists are not precisely certain just how lecithin works in the human body. However, the chief point of complete agreement brought out by research is this: *Lecithin, a by-product of the versatile soybean, does help to disperse deposits of fatty materials and reduce cholesterol in certain vital organs of the human body.*

Fortunately, lecithin comes in several forms. However, the most popular version is the granule because it is easy to sprinkle on salads, vegetables or meat dishes. Next in acceptance is the capsule because it can be swallowed easily and is quickly assimulated into the body processes.

THE AMAZING STORY OF
HOW D.W. REGAINED HIS
HEALTH AND MOBILITY

The first time I ever saw this man (we'll identify him as D.W.) he was shuffling into my class in Better Living at the Institute of Lifetime Learning, barely able to walk, even with the aid of two stout canes. Obviously, moving around was painful for him. I might state that I usually open each series of new classes with the story of how I developed my Better Living program, and I recount with enthusiasm what the program has done for me. During the presentation I make it quite clear that I do not have the slightest idea of how *my plan* of consuming natural foods will benefit someone else. All I know are the positive miracle results that I have been able to achieve.

One day after I finished my account, D.W. asked if he could tell his story. By his voice, and the way he made his plea, I knew that he was plainly reaching out for help. "About two years ago," he began, "I found that it was increasingly difficult for me to walk. Even at night my legs were paining me constantly — especially when I was trying to get some badly needed rest. Up to this point I have tried everything, including instructions from our family doctor, but nothing seems to work. Frankly, I haven't a great deal of faith in the program that helped you, Mr. Hill, especially the part about lecithin, but I'm going to give it an honest try, starting today."

When class convened the following week, I certainly wasn't prepared for what I saw. D.W. walked into the room, almost briskly and took his usual seat with an air of confidence that was a joy to behold. When all was quiet D.W. again asked if he could say a few words. Without any preliminaries he told the following story: "Your lecture last week was the greatest thing that has ever happened to me. I'll admit I followed the program you outlined with some misgivings at first, but after only two days my improvement was so marked that I began to take a new lease on life. Within another week I know I will be back in the swing of things. My thanks will be forever yours."

All of this happened five years ago. Yesterday afternoon I encountered D.W. on the street. He was swinging along, almost gaily when he saw me. "Hi," he greeted with a big, broad grin. "Tomorrow I'll be celebrating my eighty-fifth birthday — and I'm getting more out of life than I did at fifty — and I know it's because I listened to what I thought at the time was your way-out lecture. Believe me, I am more than grateful for your suggestions." And with that he was off, but quickly added, "I want to get to the sporting goods store before they close."

HEALTHFUL SOY FLOUR
CAN BE MADE FROM SOYBEANS

Among health-minded persons, the consumption of bread made from soybean flour is increasing steadily. This is true, not only because of the valuable lecithin content of soy flour, but also because of its high nutritional qualities. At one time bread made from soy flour could only be purchased in the more progressive health food stores. As knowledge of the nutritional qualities of soy flour spreads, an ever-increasing number of grocery stores now carry the *soya staff of life*. This trend seems to have every indication of growing. In small baked items such as biscuits and cookies, lecithin is able to produce a dough that is much drier. Stickiness is greatly lessened. This advantage alone is quite helpful in production and marketing.

PRODUCTION OF LECITHIN IS INCREASING STEADILY

Lecithin, now available for use in commerce, is produced at an annual rate of close to 150 million pounds. Obviously, the outlook for increasing use of soybean lecithin is definitely encouraging. In fact, ready-for-use poundage figures should build up substantially within the next decade. Every day more and more persons are learning of the real merit of lecithin as an aid to extending the life span.

For example, production of lecithin has a yearly increase well over 20 million pounds — occurring in less than a quarter of a century. This is an amazing record of growth. During the past twenty-five years, output has passed the 60-million-pound mark — causing an influx of the golden granules into the health food stores across the nation at a steady pace. Most of this fantastic gain is caused because of its acceptance as an aid to better health.

At this time a good grade of lecithin sells in health food stores for somewhere in the neighborhood of $6 for a 16-ounce package. Naturally enough, this wide spread between the price paid to processors and the cost to the consumer seems to be inordinately high. When the time comes that competition will force the price to a reasonable figure, I am convinced the market will absorb ten times the present volume. With this strong marketing situation going for them, the health food stores should find the sale of all of their other products increasing. When prices go too high it limits sales and is certainly not sound business profit-wise.

THE SUBSTANCE WITH
A WIDE VARIETY OF FOOD USES

Within the broad picture, prospects for lecithin derived from soybeans is unusually promising. As acreage devoted to cultivating soybeans increases, prices to the consumer should become more realistic. When this happens the whole economy will be benefited.

Commercial grades of lecithin are used in ever-widening variety of food products. Clearly, the purpose is to achieve maximum emulsification of fats. There is also another valid reason why bakers include lecithin in nearly all baked goods. Consistency of the salable product is greatly improved. Appearance and eating qualities are increased at comparatively very small cost. The finished product is more appetizing. With this real benefit to retailers in evidence, the big push is on. Among other advantages, lecithin is an antioxident. This means shelf life is extended for the various products.

It is now established that lecithin is both nutritious and wholesome as a food. Lecithin possesses certain important elements that play an essential role in metabolism.

Good quality grades of lecithin are classified by the Food and Drug Administration as GRAS. Translated, this means: *generally recognized as safe.*

At this time many food-producing operations in all parts of the country are using soybeans or soybean products because of the high protein content. Naturally enough, producers are also strongly motivated because profits are greater. Cost-conscious school lunch operators and public institutions of all kinds use this new food whenever possible, and it is used in many eating establishments where health is considered important. This acceptance of lecithin as a valuable food product points in one direction only—a respected place in the production and distribution of foods.

More and more persons are faced with preparing meals for away-from-home consumption. Soybeans, with their long-lasting freshness, plus high protein values, plus the healthful benefits of their lecithin content are ideal for foods prepared well in advance of eating.

PRODUCTION OF
THE EMULSIFYING SUBSTANCE
SKYROCKETS

Lecithin was discovered and used long before soybeans became popular. Before it was learned how to produce lecithin from soybeans, the only source of this valuable product was egg yolks. Prices for the food grade of lecithin used to range from $25 to $35 per pound. Obviously, this made use of the substance prohibitive for bakers and candy makers. When the processed soybean emerged on the American market as a new source of lecithin, new and more sophisticated techniques for separating lecithin from the beans were soon developed. As a consequence, wholesale prices in the open market at one time dropped as low as 15 cents per pound for good grades.

After this unpretentious beginning, venturesome men began to probe for more of the secrets of soybeans. When it was revealed that one small part of the soybean possessed a product that would emulsify fats, commercial uses for this part blossomed all over the place. This derivative of the new farm crop literally opened *Pandora's box* for at least seven major industries. They were: health foods, candy making, baking, paint, the food service market, a wide variety of manufacturing uses, and in the blending of margarines. Some record for one part of a tiny bean!

It is difficult to believe that from a modest beginning — less than a century ago — the annual planting of soybeans in the United States now exceeds 50 million acres.

When this announcement was made recently by the U.S. Department of Agriculture, the statement was met with open incredulity. "It is simply impossible," declared one farm expert. But the fact remains, the production of this versatile crop is growing by *leaps and bounds*. And all for many excellent reasons. Chief among the causes for this explosion of interest were the health food fadists who had discovered the tremendous benefits to be gained by sprinkling lecithin granules, one of the forms of this versatile product, over salads, in soups, stews and sauces. The avowed purpose was to reduce blood cholesterol. From all of the accounts I can gather, this belief was valid.

In one of my class groups, a lady, whom we shall call Estelle V., had been told by her doctor that her blood cholesterol was 325 and her blood pressure was 190 over 120, and she had an advanced case of arteriosclerosis (hardening of the arteries). She had been put on a very strict diet, but she was still uneasy about her health. When she heard our discussion about the claims made for lecithin, she decided to give it a try. Six weeks later, when she went in for a blood count, her cholesterol had dropped to 275 and her blood pressure had dropped to 180 over 110. To say that she was elated over her improvement would be putting it mildly. From that point on, her gains were quite steady and she happily informed the class that a recent examination showed that her cholesterol count was down to 240, her blood pressure was down to 150 over 90, and hardening of her arteries seemed to be greatly reduced. She seemed thoroughly convinced that it was because she sprinkled lecithin on much of the food she consumed.

WHY IS LOW CHOLESTEROL IMPORTANT?

While it is true that cholesterol is important in metabolism, it is nonetheless a body product that is known to cause *arteriosclerosis*. When a person finds he has that problem he learns that too much cholesterol will cause hardening of the walls of the arteries in a manner that makes circulation of the blood extremely difficult. Up to this time, there is apparently only one natural product we know that is capable of dissolving these harmful deposits—lecithin. While it is true that some drugs have been developed that are helpful, the side effects are still unknown. Any product that is taken for this purpose should only be used under competent medical supervision.

STARTLING RESULTS REVEALED

During my research on this subject, I was able to interview over one hundred persons who had used lecithin for a variety of accepted physical ailments. Consensus was almost eighty percent favorable. Responses ranged all the way from little or no benefit to a definite improvement in general health. One eighty-two-year-old man, who was barely able to shuffle around, was up and fully active again in less than two weeks. I am sure similar situations can be found by any researcher willing to probe for facts.

During the seven years that I taught the principles of Better Living to large and enthusiastic classes, I observed great improvement among my students and those to whom I told the lecithin story. As its beneficial effects become better known, I have been trying to find out the reasons for the favorable action of lecithin on health and why it helps to relieve so many different human ills. Since so little is now known by the present medical profession about lecithin and its action on the human body, I would like to record what I have found out. It must be understood that this is my own information gathered from many sources and researching great volumes of material that does not have the approval of medical doctors at this time. The findings that I have described are my own. There is still much controlled testing to be done, but it should be accomplished by persons willing to accept the results of such investigations.

There is a variety of lecithins derived from various sources, but they do not vary in composition to any very great extent. All types contain approximately the same elements. The best known lecithin is probably the one derived from the lowly bean and not from egg yolk. So much needs to be learned about this versatile product, as I have previously stated.

Lecithin is a very large and yet compact molecule of organic matter, containing both phosphoric acid and choline. This molecule is also a vitamin, a vitamin that regulates the deposition of fats in the liver as one of its main functions. An important part of lecithin contains a vitamin called inositol which is essential to life.

All of the functions of this vitamin are not yet known, but it does seem to be required for the health of the skin and hair. Inositol is found in minute amounts in all the cells of the body. It is ten times as abundant in the human body as any other vitamin except nicotinic acid. It is hard to understand why, unless inositol is of great value in human physiology, it should be present in such large amounts.

A HIGH-PROTEIN BEVERAGE
OF GROWING POPULARITY

In nearly all areas of the world, food shortages are increasing because of a rapidly increasing population. The "population explosion" is not only critical because it strains other resources, but because it is devouring diminishing food supplies. We must find ways to slow down population growth throughout the world and at the same time find new food sources.

Reducing world population growth is complicated because some shallow-minded religionists refuse to allow birth control. Attention therefore turns to finding new food sources, and to make use of such substances as soybean by-products.

Unfortunately, the lessening production of milk means that supplies of dry milk solids are steadily declining. The only answer at this time appears to be a protein beverage made from soybeans. "Soy milk" is gaining in acceptance in the U.S., and many foreign countries are getting the idea.

Within the past two years the Northern Regional Research Laboratory, located in Peoria, Illinois, has developed a new process for using extruded full-fat soy flour for the preparation of a spray-dried product suitable for making a highly nutritious beverage.

When the flour is reconstituted with water, a flavorful milk is produced. Cost of making this new *milk* is roughly estimated to be less than 25 cents per gallon. This figure is based upon the going price of soybeans. Clearly enough this brings an extremely palatable and nourishing beverage within range of everybody's pocketbook.

Vera G., for example, was allergic to cow's milk in the sense that all she did was gain unwanted weight without really satisfying her appetite. In fact, she seemed to be hungry all the time and the more pounds she put on the hungrier she became. Her energy was decreasing to the point where she was tired most of the time. When she heard of the new "milk" product made from soybeans, she decided to give it a whirl. The results were little short of fantastic. She began losing weight. Her worktime energy was picking up by the day. Within three months she was like a person reborn. She had lost forty pounds of ugly fat and instead of dragging around all day at her job she was so full of pep that she was soon promoted to a more responsible position. To Vera, at least, a high protein beverage was an answer to a sincere prayer.

THOUGHTS ABOUT
THE THIRD MAGIC SECRET

(1) Lecithin, a source of phosphorous, inositol, and choline, all needed by the body, is the magic ingredient in soybeans.
(2) Soybeans contain many other valuable nutrients.
(3) Lecithin is known to control cholesterol and reduce the likelihood of arteriosclerosis.
(4) A milk substitute has been made from soybeans that is a wonderfully nutritious high-protein drink.

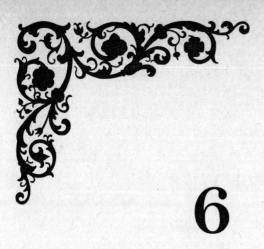

6

THE FOURTH
MAGIC HEALTH SECRET:
HEALING POWER IN AN
EASILY GROWN GARDEN PLANT

With a few exceptions, the only real benefit to come to us out of all the drug laboratories are the family of *antibiotics*, including the familiar penicillin, and the group of preparations developed from disease germs and known as *vaccines*. We must admit that these results of laboratory research have wiped out some of the worst afflictions haunting mankind.

Now, however, the developers of new drugs seem to push ahead so far that they are reaching for the moon. Why should they strive so hard to find new healing substances when nature

has provided us with all of the healing substances we need —
non-drug products that do not bring on harmful or dangerous
side effects.

THE WONDERFUL REMEDY

It is always fascinating to look at some of the old time
home remedies, which are passed from one generation to another, and discover how only the ones that are truly effective
pass the test of time. I am, of course, referring to one in particular: comfrey. The leaves of this plant have been used for
centuries as an effective demulcent and astringent.

Today medical science is taking a second look at this old-
time herbal remedy. In his book, "Russian Comfrey", the
British writer Lawrence D. Hills refers to allantoin, the active
therapeutic agent found so abundantly in this remarkable
plant, comfrey, as an internal healer.

Recently, my son, Bob, suffered a badly broken ankle in a
freak street accident. After a thorough examination of numerous X-rays, he was informed that he would have to wear the cast
for at least six weeks, but the toughest blow of all was the pronouncement by the doctor that he should not return to work for
six months. Even though he was fully covered by insurance, he
was really up-tight over this ruling. Bob had often heard me
mention the apparently magic healing properties of comfrey
and at this point he was willing to try anything. He purchased a
bottle of comfrey tablets at the local health food store and followed the directions on the label to the letter. Within three
days all pain had disappeared. For some obscure reason it was
necessary to change the cast for additional X-rays. Much to the
doctor's amazement, the "break" was obviously healed. One

week later, Bob was back on the job "as good as new." Several months have now passed with no problems in evidence.

H. E. Kirschner, M.D., describes comfrey in his book, "Nature's Healing Grasses." He used it in his practice and in his book he reports some case histories of patients in which comfrey was used in cases involving open wounds, burns, insect bites, gastric ulcers, lung ailments and internal tumors.

Dr. Kirschner writes, "As a blood purifier, comfrey has been widely used in European countries for centuries, and is highly recommended in old medical books and herbals. The Europeans cooked the leaves and ate them as we do spinach or beet greens."

It is interesting to learn that the healing agent, allantoin, is present in both the roots and the leaves of comfrey, and its value as a cell-proliferant — in making the edges of wounds grow together, healing sores, and taken internally for gastric and duodenal ulcers, and intestinal irritations causing diarrhea — is still recognized in pharmacy.

"By the way," Dr. Kirschner went on to say, "comfrey is very easy to grow in the backyard. It just needs good soil and water."

MIRACLE MENDING POWERS

Plants for medicinal purposes, of which comfrey is but one of many, are truly remarkable. Down through the centuries herbs have served the rich and the poor, the sick and the lame. Today their healing qualities are still available to those who will take the time to search.

Among the vast array of herbs and grasses that we know, comfrey stands tall as a healing agent. It is helpful, not only in

its mending powers, but is is remarkably effective as a demulcent and an astringent. In its natural state, comfrey seems to
flourish best in moist, warm, and low-ground areas. The plant
is a member of the Borage family of herbs.

It is known that a thousand years before Christ the ancient
Greeks were using comfrey. In fact, it was included in the very
earliest knowledge of medicinal herbs. During Elizabethan
times, herbalist Culpepper listed comfrey as one of the most
effective natural healing agents.

POWER OF THE
CELL PROLIFERANT

Comfrey is just an ordinary salad-green type of plant, but
it has proved to contain an unusual substance that is quite
helpful in many ways. It has been variously described as a tonic,
a blood builder, and as possessing unusual qualities in stimulating new tissue growth. What else could one ask for in a product
of nature?

A very special quality that provides this lowly herb with
its claim to fame derives from one ingredient — *allantoin,* a
cell proliferant. This special property of the comfrey leaf can
do so many things for the human body that it would be difficult
to enumerate them here without stretching your credulity. Suffice to say that it is actually one of the wonder products of
nature's bounty.

For example, a few years ago my doctor, an extremely
competent person for an M.D., diagnosed the excruciating pain
in my joints as *degenerative rhumatoid arthritis.* A trip to the
X-ray specialist confirmed his opinion. What to do now? About
all the good doctor could offer was a prescription for a high-
priced pain-killer. Because the situation was critical for me, I

developed a great interest in the products of nature. A trip to the health food store revealed a great reservoir of information covering the topic of herbs. In one of the little books offered for sale I found one about comfrey. So many remarkable things had happened to persons who had eaten the magic green plant that I decided to give the product a try. Within three days the pain in my joints began to lessen and within a few weeks I was feeling like a new person. It was at this point that I began a serious study of nature's own healers.

At first my doctor friend took a very dim view of my self-help program — in fact he even quipped, "A person who doctors himself has a fool for a patient." Today, though, my continued health speaks for itself.

What will comfrey do for *you?* Truthfully, I haven't the slightest idea. All I can do is point to the record — derived from the many letters and reports that come to me, plus my own research on the subject.

I realize now that some of my discoveries must have seemed sheer stupidity to a highly-trained medical man, but I refused to accept a lifetime of suffering as final. At my time of life, which is well past the proverbial *three-score-and ten,* I am living life to the hilt. Among other things I recently returned from a cross-country trip in order to keep a lecture engagement. I welcome more of these opportunities to appear on both radio and TV talk shows.

EXTERNAL USE AS A POULTICE

During the many years in which I developed class discussions and research on comfrey, I gathered notes that are constant reminders. For instance, comfrey may be used as a poultice. Hard-to-heal sores, insect bites, and open wounds have responded favorably, according to persons I have interviewed.

Comfrey is used as one of the special ingredients in cosmetics and is claiming some remarkable demonstrations. For example, it is soothing and tends to overcome ordinary skin irritations. It does possess some remarkable qualities as a skin softener — especially when dry or chapped conditions prevail.

Comfrey also has an unusual reputation for eliminating ordinary skin spots. I have tried it with startling results. I had to have four "blemishes" removed (prior to the time I knew of comfrey) by painful cutting, and even worse, long-drawn-out X-ray treatments. Now when a spot is "suspect" I use a small poultice of comfrey powder softened with a drop of liquid chlorophyll and the threatening red spot disappears within a very few days.

Comfrey mixed with other nutrients can double their efficiency. I have found that when I pour a tablespoonful of strong comfrey tea into my chlorophyll and orange juice cocktail before breakfast, I am well prepared for the day's work.

Comfrey as a tea is developing a good reputation as an internal healer. This includes such stubborn afflictions as gastric ulcers. Ask your physician, and if he doesn't object, try comfrey tea.

Don't make the mistake of regarding comfrey as an herb that is good for everything — a "cure all." Without any doubt the leaves of this versatile plant do possess some important healing qualities. Nearly all of the so-called miracle results that comfrey has achieved comes from its one claim to fame — allantoin. It is also noteworthy that each of the magic secrets of long life has a secret ingredient or some very special quality. Which of these unique attributes will take care of your particular need is a question that only you can answer.

AN IMPRESSIVE
HISTORY OF HEALING

It is known that comfrey has been used as a healer since the dawn of history. Before the time of written records, it seems reasonable to assume that early types of *homo sapiens* knew about the healing qualities of this particular plant. Little wonder that this commonplace herb has won for itself a niche in the annals of folk medicine.

Should you elect to try comfrey for any purpose, you should know one outstanding advantage in its use: It combines exceedingly well when the dried leaves are mixed with simple beverages or eaten with other foods. I mean you can add it to fresh fruit or vegetable juices or mix it in salads. It is especially compatible with the juice of the fresh alfalfa plant, which is better known as chlorophyll.

STANDING TALL
IN FOOD VALUES

Luckily for the human race, inquiring minds survived the artificial wisdom brought on by the Victorian years. With the coming of the twentieth century, once again open minds began to reassess the works of earlier physicians. This probing into the mysteries of nature soon revealed proof of what had formerly been nothing more than folk remedies. With the advent of improved testing procedures it was soon discovered that in addition to the healing power of *allantoin*, this precious plant comfrey possessed some vitamins and important trace minerals. This was apparently true because roots of the comfrey plant bore deeply into subsoil for nourishment.

When you begin to add up all of the known healing qualities of comfrey, it seems safe to assume that a good cup of strong comfrey tea is precisely what the doctor should prescribe — instead of drugs of doubtful quality, or worse, drugs capable of causing harmful side-effects.

The original author of *Materia Medica,* Dioscorides, noted first century botanist and physician, mentioned the fact that comfrey was favorably known for its healing qualities — externally for wounds, and internally for its ability to aid in helping bones to knit rapidly. With this sort of recognition, herbalists of the Middle Ages described its merits in the medical treatises.

Unfortunately, in the early years of the nineteenth century "learned" doctors were prone to scoff at the healing powers of comfrey as so much nonsense. If it hadn't been for more knowledgable peasant women who kept right on maintaining the family health with comfrey, this valuable herb might have been lost to us. (In this connection, note that early settlers in America fed comfrey leaves to sick farm animals with remarkably favorable results.)

YOU CAN GROW YOUR OWN

Your own introduction to medicinal herbs, can be as close as your backyard. Right there, just a few short steps from your back door, you can plant a miniature herb garden that will be as useful and educational as it is helpful.

All you really need is a small area of only a few feet in an area that gets plenty of sunshine. The soil doesn't have to be especially fertile — most herbs are hardy "weeds" that can survive under Spartan conditions — but it should at least be well-drained. And keep your plot free of real weeds so that your fledgling plants can grow and thrive.

Once again, one of the distinct advantages of comfrey derives from the fact that the plant can easily be grown in your own garden or window box. All you have to do is go to your reliable health food store and purchase starting roots. Some of the more up-to-date places carry partly grown plants ready and waiting for you to start your own source of a valuable health food. All you need is two or three starter plants and you will soon have enough of the large rough leaves to be used fresh in your salads, stews, or soups. Or you can dry the leaves and powder them to mix with other foods or you can make your own tea. When dried, the leaves are easily stored for the time when you need them. There are about twenty-five to thirty varieties that can be used as a tea in any strength that suits your taste.

Comfrey, one of the most helpful of the nine magic secrets, has one more important advantage. You can take a tablet, the powder, or even a few dried leaves to make an efficient poultice. Should you have a *trouble spot* show up any place in or on your body, it won't hurt to try comfrey. It is completely non-toxic. But if you are at all suspicious about the spot, check with your family doctor, before using comfrey.

It is really unfortunate that the medical profession has given too little attention to the healing qualities of herbs. All too many doctors are so deeply concerned with modern *miracle drugs* that simple remedies of the past are often overlooked. A few enlightened doctors, however, have interested themselves in herbs with good "word-of-mouth" reputations. Some medical doctors have even gone so far as to grow some of the better-known varieties in properly composted soil—*free of chemical fertilizers, or poisonous pesticides.*

HERBAL HEALING —
AN ANCIENT ART

When the art of healing the sick was in its infancy, ancient man had only the products of nature to mend his ills. It was in this fashion that folk lore began to attach certain benefits to this or that type of herb. Gradually "medicine men" evolved from this process — persons who specialized in *knowing* what each herb would do for the user. The "herbal healers" helped many, and still do. Their somewhat hit-or-miss type of prescribing, however, brought the caustic comment from one doctor who specializes in internal medicine, "It is a dangerous throwback to the Middle Ages."

Soon laws were passed preventing use of herbal medicines, as the *bureaucrats* jumped on their little hobby-horses and declared, "They can kill." Just *what* they would kill hasn't been made quite clear in any of the so-called learned circles. Should competent testing reveal that disease germs would be the ones to suffer demise, the ill-advised remarks would be worthwhile.

I have tried to determine the source of all this anti-herb propaganda. Obviously, much of the bigotry and hate teachings derive from poorly informed persons, or worse, men and women committed to the vast chemical industries. Without question, no one should eat, drink, or take any drug, herb, or watery concoction without competent advice—*given in truth*. Anything less is deceptive and lacking in common sense.

Certainly the public is entitled to know the facts about all products offered for sale—especially those items processed, manufactured, or grown, that foster claims of great therapeutic value. Perhaps it is well that peoples of the world are being aroused to the fact that the medical profession is not infallable. Now we should know the truth about the curative qualities of certain leaves, roots, berries, bark, and perhaps flowers—

particularly those which seem to provide extremely important trace minerals—the bureaucrats to the contrary notwithstanding.

Some herbs seem to help counteract drug addition. Young persons suckered into taking drugs as a means of escape from reality, are finding a way back with herbs. Exactly which herb will do the job is open to debate. Some have found relief and/or release from the habit with ginseng. Others have added chlorophyll. A few have included lecithin, and a lesser number are drinking a variety of herb teas. Should anyone you know suffer from a terrible drug affliction have him/her see a *competent* medical doctor first. *It is the law.* When the drug addict's medical advisor agrees, the afflected person can seek help from herbs. Some persons who have recovered from addiction regularly use herbs. Many of the victims will gladly supply you with *tried and true* means of finding a *way out.*

Wouldn't it be far better for trained researchers to probe the verity of this antidote?

In wrapping up this particular discussion, should you find yourself in real trouble with drugs, or even suspect you have a problem, seek the help of a *competent* medical man or woman — as quickly as possible.

THOUGHTS ABOUT
THE FOURTH MAGIC SECRET

(1) For centuries people have used various herbs to heal illnesses.

(2) Comfrey, one of the most versatile members of the herb family, may be applied either internally or externally, and possesses an almost endless variety of health uses.

(3) Do not think of comfrey as a "cure-all," but consider
     ways in which it can benefit you.
(4) Medical practitioners are now taking a closer look at
     the advantages comfrey seems to have.
(5) Fresh comfrey leaves make excellent additions to
     salads, soups, stews and sauces.

7

THE FIFTH
MAGIC HEALTH SECRET:
THE WONDERFUL CORNERSTONE
OF LONG LIFE

An ever-increasing number of medical researchers and scientists are beginning to suspect that vitamin E can slow down the aging process and extend an active life-span by as much as thirty years.

In support of this startling bit of evidence are the laboratory experiments now being conducted by Dr. Lester Packer and James R. Smith of the University of California. Human body cells have been kept alive in a laboratory culture for one-and-a-half times longer than normal when a small amount of vitamin E was added to the test-tube mixture. I believe exhaustive testing procedures should be applied to this vitamin at once. For example, one powerful organization, The Heart Association, should be asked to make tests of vitamin E.

A VITAMIN THAT SEEMS TO PREVENT HEART ATTACKS

At this time considerable evidence is accumulating in favor of the restorative qualities of vitamin E in overcoming many common diseases. No one seems to know precisely how vitamin E brings about the effect it produces. It is now claimed that many miraculous "cures" have been achieved by creative medical doctors—especially when vitamin E has been added to the diet of ailing patients.

One point is worthy of note: Proponents assert that persons who consume vitamin E regularly almost without exception, rarely suffer heart attacks or similar physical disabilities.

Should you be suffering from heart disease, you are probably under the care of a medical doctor. The chances are about nine-to-one that vitamin E is not being prescribed for you. Should this be true, ask your doctor, "Why not?"—for it has now been proved conclusively that vitamin E is non toxic, produces no side effects, and there is an excellent chance that you will be greatly helped.

Now is the time to establish facts about treatment so that the truth about vitamin E will emerge. To begin with, let us frankly admit that vitamin E is greatly over-sold in a few instances by overly-zealous advertising and quite often the product is over-priced. However, the clear, unmistakable fact remains that persons who consume products high in vitamin E are enjoying good health. This is especially noticeable when the other foods they eat possess equal nutritional qualities. For example, everybody quotes Dr. Shute. Whenever the subject of vitamin E is tossed into the conversation among knowledgeable persons, the name of Evan V. Shute, Medical Director of The Shute Institute for Clinical and Laboratory Medicine, located in London, Canada, is the most quoted authority.

For nearly half a century this enterprising researcher has been testing and extolling the virtues of vitamin E, not only in his private practice, but also in his lectures, articles of scientific journals, exhibits, and in the presentation of case histories. Unfortunately, much of his prodigious work was ignored in the United States until recently.

Vitamin E is either the health bonanza it is claimed to be, or its vaunted merits should be limited to the statement made by Dr. Chute in a recent TV interview: "Vitamin E reduces the need for oxygen."

Fortunately for all of us, Dr. Shute plunged right on with his research, documentation and experiments in spite of the ridicule heaped upon him by his contemporaries. At long last he is gaining recognition for his discoveries.

Worldwide research continues to pile up in support of the advantages of taking Vitamin E. For example, in Haifa, Israel, Prof. David Gershon, working with his scientific team at the Technion Institute of Technology, reports that they have lengthened the life of laboratory animals by up to 30 percent with Vitamin E. Apparently this valuable product tends to slow down the oxidation of cells, one of the main causes of aging.

Meanwhile, American scientists are at work evaluating and updating the minimum daily requirements for Vitamin E. The latest to suggest supplementing the diet with this vitamin is M. D. Horwitt, Ph.D., professor of biochemistry at St. Louis University School of Medicine. He reviews, favorably, the development of adult daily needs in an article in a recent issue of the American Journal of Clinical Nutrition.

THE PROPER AMOUNT
YOU SHOULD TAKE

It is obvious that a massive intake of vitamin E, without your doctor's approval could be risky. At this time far-ranging claims are gaining in acceptance that this unusual vitamin will prevent certain physical ailments. Some investigators assert that vitamin E will retard the aging process, restore sexual potency, and shield us against air pollution. Hopefully, all this is true. However, it is known worldwide that men and women are consuming vitamin E tablets and capsules in ever-increasing quantities. Naturally enough, suppliers are pleased.

John S. from Indiana, told me he suffered a moderate heart attack, After six weeks in the hospital his doctor advised him not to work for at least the next six months and to lose thirty pounds at the very minimum, otherwise he would have a small chance of survival.

Losing weight wasn't too much of a problem, but John S. found loafing intolerable. Quite by chance he happened to hear one of my radio talk shows in which I told of the experiments under way with vitamin E with heart patients. Willing to try anything, John sought out his local drug store and purchased a bottle of the highest potency Vitamin E he could get. Results didn't seem exactly miraculous, but three weeks later he was feeling so much better that he made an appointment with his doctor for a check-up. In John's words, "The man of medicine was so astonished by my improvement that he 'allowed as how' I could go back to work."

According to drugstore operators and health food store owners, the sale of vitamin E has increased amazingly during the past twelve years. When the smoke of controversy over the merits of vitamin E clears away, it is hoped we can get to the truth. It is our purpose within this book to separate fact from fancy. For example, the majority of doctors insist that we are getting all of the E we require in our food, providing we are eating a balanced diet. A "balanced diet" for one person, however, may not serve someone else's individual need.

On the other hand, health food store operators and thoughtful nutritionists, along with a few open-minded medical practitioners, see a potential of merit in a reasonable intake of vitamin E. This is the other point of view.

Personally I take 800 units a day. However, I cannot prescribe for you. You'll have to determine your own body needs by consulting your family doctor or by your reaction to this valuable natural food.

Many of us have been denied a rich source of vitamin E ever since flour began to be machine-milled. Well over a century ago, our free enterprise system erred grieviously in favor of taste and convenience. This occurred when an inventor created the high-speed-roller-mill to be used in the milling of flour. The result of milling flour with this new device was to remove the bran and wheat germ which was rich in vitamin E from the seed. When this happened, the bright geniuses of the early establishment described these left-overs as offals.

The fallacies imposed upon us long ago become absurd when it is known that these same offals are considered valuable for feeding farm animals but when used for human consumption are of little value. Why do the bureaucrats claim such a vast difference? It simply doesn't make sense.

WHAT THIS AMAZING VITAMIN REALLY IS

From a strictly chemical description, E is composed of a group of several substances represented as *tocopherols*. Source of this important material derives mostly from grains and vegetable oils. Other foods contain E in varying amounts, mostly small. Certainly not enough to contribute any great benefit to your desire for long life.

In my classes at the Institute of Lifetime Learning, I present both sides of the vitamin E controversy. Some persons accept the favorable opinions as valid, while others go along with the beliefs of the *status quo* proponents. The men and women who have added vitamin E to their daily intake of food are in reasonably good health. All but one of those who rejected the idea have passed on, to use a polite euphemism.

My experience in matters of research is limited to a group of about five hundred mentally active persons. Most of them are retired. Why not expand this limited testing to include all ages, with all manner of health problems? This procedure might produce amazing answers good for the improved health of the nation. It is your right to know the real truth.

Since the "vitamin gold-rush" burst upon the American scene shortly after World War II ended, much controversy has raged over this single health product, vitamin E.

What does this mean to the men and women in search of a better life? About all we can offer at this time is a close look at the record.

SOME CLAIMS
NOT YET PROVED

Vitamin E needs a champion. The late Adelle Davis, noted author and health lecturer, was one of the few articulate defenders of vitamin E. Obviously, more men and women of Mrs. Davis' character and courage are needed now. This is true for the plain reason that many of the way-out claims for its merits have yet to be disproved.

Clearly enough this is not a valid reason to fight progress. In my opinion (and I have taken pains to evaluate both sides of the issue) there is more than a grain of truth in the claims made by backers of vitamin E and less than a grain of truth in the claims coming from opponents.

How am I so sure of my position? From personal experience, and from the reports coming to me from hundreds of persons who have attended my lectures. In all instances, I have asked for honest answers. In telling the story of vitamin E I state very carefully that "Here is what the pro's say about the worth of vitamin E and here is the position of the con's."

What about burns? In this connection, my own experience is limited. Recently, while preparing a meal over an open camp fire, a splatter of hot grease caused a bad burn on my arm. The pain was excruciating. A quick search of my first aid kit revealed nothing helpful except a bottle of vitamin E capsules. I bit one open and spread the oil over the burn. Instantly, the pain was relieved. Afterward, healing was much more rapid than usual. Later, when I recounted my experience to my class, several persons reported similar results.

Incredible as it might appear at first glance, it is now maintained that the versatile E is an excellent deodorant. Who is it that makes this assertion? An old and respected cosmetic company!

There was a full-page ad appearing recently in a national magazine which featured this new use of vitamin E. Among other statements made, it was admitted that the scientific community is at long last focusing its attention on the merits of this natural product. And for apparently very good reason. Serious research by the company is now attempting to unlock the full potential of vitamin E, with the result that this long ignored vitamin is now claiming a new benefit. Reason for its effectiveness, according to the manufacturer, derives from the simple fact that the action is antioxident in nature. This claim I find difficult to accept.

Treatment with vitamin E for any one of the ills of human-kind is elementary and comparatively inexpensive. Until recently prices were high, when this product of nature was only available in health food stores. Now such giant firms as the Squibb company, are distributing high-quality vitamin E at lower prices to all drugstores.

"GROWING OLD STOPPED COLD"
DECLARES ONE NOTED RESEARCHER

In presenting the role vitamin E plays in regard to aging, Dr. Erwin Di Cyan clearly states: "I believe that vitamin E slows down the process of aging so that taking it in sufficient daily amounts can possibly make a person of 60 look, act, feel, *seem* and *be* more like a person of 50, or a person of 70 look, act, feel, seem to be more like a person of, say, 60..."

Now is the time to get down to facts so that the truth about vitamin E will emerge.

THOUGHTS ABOUT
THE FIFTH MAGIC SECRET

(1) Vitamin E appears to have excellent healing properties, but its actions need further scientific investigation.

(2) Dr. Shute, of London, Canada, has reported excellent health results with this vitamin. Now is the time his findings should be checked.

(3) You should not hesitate to use this vitamin if you find it helpful to you.

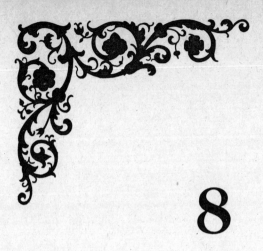

8

THE SIXTH
MAGIC HEALTH SECRET:
STRANGE EFFECTS OF
AN UNUSUAL ROOT

During the Korean War, when Russia was allied with China, the Chinese and North Korean forces managed to harvest and ship more than 20 million dollars' worth of the valuable ginseng root to Vladivostok in Russia. It was at this point the Russian scientists began to make a serious study of ginseng. A determined effort was made to discover the beneficial qualities of the root and its apparent healing effects on the human body.

Every fall an unusual breed of hunter is combing the Appalachia's hills and hollows, but instead of guns, they are carrying shovels. The questing folk are seeking a five-leafed plant with bright, red berries. Some of them may want to eat their quarry on the spot, but most of them would rather sell their find to eager buyers.

They're after *ginseng*, widely known as the "magic root."

At this time the root is selling for $60 a pound and, naturally, quite a few persons are out digging for the elusive root according to S. D. Fuller.

Another report comes from Jim Olson. He says that "You have to dig about three pounds of it this time of year to get a pound by the time it's dried. See that root over there on the wall?" he went on to explain, "the big one shaped like a carrot? Well, when I found it, it weighed ten ounces. Now it has dried out to about two ounces." The popular name for ginseng is "sang." This root doesn't like the sun. Olson continued to say that "It seems to thrive better in shady hollows in acid soil. Usually near oak trees. These roots are sent to New York periodically and are purchased mostly by Chinese agents who ship them to Hong Kong." The Chinese love ginseng. In fact, many Chinese believe it restores body vigor and stimulates the sexual organs.

Today ginseng is increasingly growing in favor in all parts of Europe. For example, one West German distributor reports his sales now exceed 60,000 bottles of the dried root every month. Demands for this strange root are growing steadily, according to the sales manager of this company.

THE HEALING FAME OF
THIS ROOT SPREADS

From the remote mountain canyons of Eastern Asia to the sophisticated European or American home is a tremendous distance in miles and cultures. However, Korean ginseng root, long known for its helpful qualities, has been used for endless centuries by Oriental peoples. Now it is finding a secure place in the American home.

Appreciation is growing for the ginseng root, but equally amazing, the traditional value of herbal remedies of the Far East is rapidly growing in popularity.

The fundamental principle of Oriental medical philosophy is that good health is a result of maintaining the dynamic balance of nature. For man this means living in harmony with the laws of nature. All of the known healing arts have the same purpose: to bring about this balance when it is upset because of a haphazard way of living. The extent of any person's imbalance will determine the special type of herbal mixture needed.

Scientists are now discovering that many of the claims for ginseng by the Chinese during past centuries can be proved. In one series of experiments on white rats, one researcher found that the animals given ginseng under strict control had far greater endurance and a longer life-span than the animals that were not fed ginseng. Other studies now in progress by an ever-increasing number of studies seem to confirm the Chinese beliefs.

Oriental legends and beliefs surrounding the healing powers of the ginseng root are endless. When coupled with the far-out claims made for ginseng as a cure-all for nearly every ill, the myths grow to fantastic proportions. This, unfortunately, has caused serious-minded scientists to steer clear of controlled testing for fear of being ridiculed by less venturesome colleagues.

What will ginseng do for you? Nothing, according to most United States pharmacologists. You may want to accept this, a strictly biased point of view. However, mature persons are willing to look at the record before making judgment.

If there is any one thing the Chinese could agree upon without referring the question to Premier Mao, it would be the miraculous benefits that can be derived from the use of ginseng. Millions upon millions of Orientals seek this bitter wrinkled root for its vaunted healing properties. The pure, untreated root sells regularly for as much as $200 a pound.

Now that American health food stores, food faddists, and cosmetic companies have "discovered" ginseng, the rush to buy this ancient restorative product of nature is on in full force. Many types of health products now include ginseng to some extent.

Why has ginseng been accepted with almost universal approval in China and just now beginning to gain acceptance in the United States? Some poorly-informed persons claim this is due to the fact that it comes from China. The age-old belief of the Chinese that the root's twisted shapes impart a miracle quality is finally catching on in Western countries.

Ginseng devotees are positive that American scientists will one day find a super-power in the lowly root. Should self-styled scientists insist upon sitting on their fat complacency instead of doing some honest research studies, the fault must lie in blind prejudice.

THIS ROOT CLAIMED
TO HEAL ARTHRITIS

There is one story I like to repeat at every opportunity. Six years ago the excruciating pain in my back and knees was diagnosed as degenerative rheumatoid arthritis, with my chances for recovery, nil. After many X-rays and further testing and examination, the doctor's opinion was confirmed. Soon, he told me I would only be able to walk with an aluminum "walker," and as for the pain, I would simply have to learn to live with it. This I did not like. When a friend of mine, a chiropractor, suggested that ginseng might be helpful, I was willing to try anything. Within three days my pain began to lessen and within three weeks I was almost back to normal. I now travel all over the country in order to keep important lecture engagements.

In my travels many persons tell me they eat one capsule or tablet of ginseng every day in order to maintain normal health. Others go for the two-a-day routine, one in the morning and one in mid-afternoon—a sort of ginseng break to replace the traditional cup of coffee—and far more effective and with a million times more beneficial results.

HISTORY OF THIS AMAZING ROOT

Merits of the ginseng root were first mentioned in the botanical literature of China over 4000 years ago. By this time the lowly root has had more written about its virtues than any other member of the family of roots. It has found wide acceptance in all South East Asian countries. It is claimed that, in many ways, ginseng has aided the health and well being of millions of far Eastern peoples. Every known disease is reputed to respond favorably to its secret magic.

For centuries, Oriental users have normally chewed the pieces of the root when occupational stresses became too great. Both the Chinese and Koreans also make tea from the dried roots.

Quite often qualities claimed for ginseng get "way out in left field," but there is one inescapable fact: there is something in the root that has great potency. Whether it is *psychosomatic* or real should be determined by competent researchers.

THE CLAIM THAT
THIS ROOT WILL
EXTEND YOUR SEX LIFE

In Oriental countries those who can pay the price use ginseng for healing body ills as well as a preventive medicine. Many users stress the fact that ginseng builds and sustains virility. This might account for the claim that men and women have been able to procreate healthy children at advanced ages. This could be possible because of the effect of ginseng upon the endocrine glands. In any event, ginseng is considered extremely valuable. It is known that at one time the Chinese sold Imperial ginseng for as much as $3,000 a pound.

One medical authority claims that ginseng evidently acts as a restorative and thus activates the entire glandular system. This, it is claimed, tends to stimulate all bodily functions. This in turn promotes a greater use of the vitamins and minerals in the food that is consumed.

PREMIUM PRICES FOR
THE WILD ROOT

Wild ginseng commands a higher price than the cultivated varieties. According to users, it is believed that the rejuvenating action of ginseng on the sex glands is due to certain radioactive substances that are absorbed from the soil. Because it is organic in origin, these radioactive qualities are beneficial. This is *unlike* strontium 90 and other inorganic fallout products.

It is assumed that the wild plant is more potent because it selects its own location and chooses the soil where the organic radioactivity is the highest. It is known that Indian medicine men in early America used wild ginseng in many of their treatments.

THE WONDER ROOT
TAKES ITS MAGIC FROM SOIL

Once again, what is ginseng? We know that the plant grows in secluded areas. It thrives only in special soil. It is claimed that the roots absorb all the valuable minerals from that soil, and it should be harvested only after seven years. In fact, there is a strong belief that the older the roots, the more potent the product. More than a thousand generations of Chinese and Koreans have steadfastly accepted the idea that ginseng has great merit as a restorative, and that it can safely be used as a remedy in a variety of bodily ills. It would be naive to declare that the Oriental peoples were basing their belief in ginseng on nothing more than on odd-ball superstitions.

THE ONLY SIDE EFFECT
IS STIMULATING

Most ginseng devotees insist that there are no side effects. However, some persons quickly discover they cannot take the American ginseng before retiring because it is too stimulating. According to some other users, on the other hand, ginseng tea tends to overcome insomnia.

MORE RESEARCH IS NEEDED

Clearly enough, many men and women have tested many varieties of ginseng. Obviously, it would be a monumental project to test all varieties. Even if the actions of each variety were known, individual differences in the physical make-up of each person ought to be taken into account. For example, it is known that fresh, full-strength ginseng is too stimulating for some persons, while others may require a more bracing effect. Each person must find for himself the most effective use of ginseng for his condition.

One Oriental businessman who has observed the effects of ginseng on his own countrymen, insists that ginseng works slowly to regenerate all bodily functions. It has proved to be helpful in chronic insomnia, and ulcers of various types seem to respond favorably. It is also great for hangovers. Some arthritis sufferers have found comforting relief. Improvement in hair growth and reversal of graying hair has been noted in some instances. However, the greatest boon of all is that broken bones heal faster, according to several persons I interviewed. In my own experience the aches and pains that I suffered disappeared rapidly.

It may be good for diabetes, but you should not substitute this for regular medical checkups by a competent physician.

THE CHINESE INSIST
IT IS A PANACEA

All Orientals insist that ginseng is a panacea. One would almost believe it is good for everything from dandruff to ingrowing toenails. But what about researchers? Will they be as enthusiastic without more probing? From all the evidence I have collected so far the answer seems to be an emphatic "yes."

THIS WONDER ROOT
IS NOT A DRUG

Ginseng is definitely not a drug. Its roots are rich in vitamins and minerals. Whether or not you can derive any benefits in its use is open to question. It may or may not be for you. There is only one way you can find out. Give it a fair trial— but avoid supply sources where you pay outrageous prices.

Some persons take one ginseng tablet or capsule a day and feel greatly benefited while others substitute a cup of ginseng tea for the morning and afternoon coffee break. Some persons insist that they feel a lift within minutes after drinking a cup of ginseng tea. Most persons do feel a pick-up soon after drinking a morning cup. Others get an almost immediate lift from taking a capsule of American ginseng.

There are many ways to use ginseng. Some persons like the concentrated powder form, others favor the capsules, while still others drink it as a tea. And the more venturesome chew the bitter root itself.

I am reminded of an extrememly spectacular incident. Carl J., while on a winter visit to California from Kansas, enrolled in one of my lecture series covering the topic of Better Living, hoping to learn of something that might relieve his rapidly deteriorating arthritic condition. At that time Carl was in his early eighties and obviously suffering from the ravages of painful arthritis. When I related my own experience with ginseng to my class, he decided to give the fabled root a try. At first he was more than skeptical of results, but within a week he was feeling better, and by the end of the month he was walking almost as spryly as a much younger man.

Recently I met Carl at a social function—a dance for senior citizens—and he was having the time of his life.

ONE SUPER VARIETY

There is one type of super ginseng known as "wild red." It is available in most health food stores. According to one authority, persons who use this product will always get good results. It can also be purchased in *tea tabs* individually wrapped in cellophane. It is claimed that the product contains a blend of 16 different types of ginseng roots — all of them with special advantages.

In addition to its other value, the brew is supposed to release 42 minerals — all with important body requirements. This tea is made by pouring a cup of boiling water over one tab. The beverage has a good flavor, although some ginseng is slightly bitter. Most people prefer a variety which is a trifle on the sweet side. No sugar has been added. The sweet variety of ginseng root is naturally sweet, consequently it is added to some mixtures in order to impart flavor.

In spite of ridicule and adverse comment, ginseng users will go on consuming well over a million pounds of all varieties annually, apparently with real benefits in evidence.

In Southern California health food stores are selling tea bags, capsules and tablets as fast as the producers and processors can package and deliver prime grade as well as low-grade forms of the product.

Naturally, an important question comes to the surface. Is all this hoopla warranted or is it merely being sold by an overly zealous imagination? The precious root is the source of a steadily growing and profitable business in the United States. Although ginseng is not easy to grow, it can be grown in many parts of the country, especially in the Midwest. Harvesters are known to earn from $40 to $50 per pound for prime quality dried roots. One of the largest of American exporters manages to ship about 35 tons annually to European countries.

Many enthusiastic ginseng users apparently believe it has superpowers. Alledgedly, it has many virtues. Among its more flamboyant merits, according to devotees, is that it is an aphrodisiac. This claim is open to question, as I have previously stated.

VAST ACREAGE
NOW BEING PLANTED

Following the Soviet experiments and findings, the demand for ginseng has increased worldwide. When Russia planted a huge section of land to ginseng in the maritime province of Siberia, the boom was on. When you consider that the ginseng plant requires considerable shade for proper growth, plus the fact that it takes six years or more for a root to mature before it is harvested, you can believe that the Russian decision was not reached without a great deal of planning and research before committing so much time and money to the project.

HOW CLOSE ARE WE
TO A PANACEA?

A. J. Gelfand, M.D., writing in *Let's Live Magazine*, accepts the idea that ginseng is the closest we can come to a panacea. Perhaps it is not a casual circumstance that it has been successfully improving the health of devotees for nearly 5000 years. However, his most startling observation is that *all* of the curative powers claimed for ginseng are apparently valid.

HEALTH BOON TO AUSTRALIANS

There are many so-called diseases which, it is claimed, will respond to a regular intake of ginseng. The Australians, who are known to be great consumers of North Korean ginseng, believe that the root helps to regulate blood pressure, to slow down arteriosclerosis, improve digestion, reduce constipation, reduce inflammation of the urinary tract, and be of remarkable help in overcoming fatigue.

Most of the ginseng sold in the American market comes through the Korean government monopoly. The price varies from a few dollars a pound for low grade "hair" or "tails" of the main root to two hundred dollars a pound for the completely matured roots.

Ginseng plant leftovers are used in preparing a variety of foods, but they have very little therapeutic value. When leftovers reach the American market, they are often ground and sold as a top quality product at cut-rate prices and the customer is shortchanged.

Some of the scrap fiber is cut from the main root and converted into "ginseng tea." The value of this tea is open to question. Real quality ginseng root powder sells from seven to twelve dollars an ounce. Should you feel that ginseng is for you, make certain that you purchase your supply from a reliable source.

VALID RESEARCH
NOW IN PROGRESS

It is well to know that valid research on ginseng is now in progress. A great deal of information is being collected and documented. We can assume that health magazines will share their findings with you so that you can decide for yourself.

However, there is one thing you should know: the FDA is less than happy with the whole enterprise. Ginseng distributors and health food stores alike are being challenged for making unfounded claims about the product. All I know for sure about the claimed magic of ginseng is my own experience. Arthritis was getting the better of me in no uncertain terms until I started using ginseng in every conceivable form. From that moment my health has improved to the point where I am able to write, travel and lecture world-wide. What the product will do for you I haven't the slightest idea, but anything with so much claimed magic going for it is worth a try.

THOUGHTS ABOUT
THE SIXTH MAGIC SECRET

(1) Most researchers seem to agree that the great value of the popular ginseng root derives from the natural vitamins and minerals that the root attracts from the soil in which it grows.

(2) Exaggerated claims for this root and over-selling of it have obviously hurt this valuable product with doctors and lay people alike.

(3) It has been established, however, that ginseng has no harmful side effects.

(4) Without any doubt, when someone drinks a cup of good ginseng tea, or takes a ginseng tablet, he is at least receiving far more dependable stimulation than when he swallows a cup of coffee.

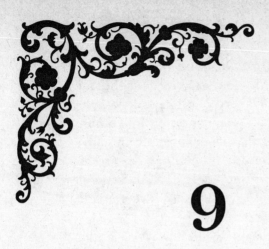

9

THE SEVENTH
MAGIC HEALTH SECRET:
HOW TO USE THE
VITAL FORCE OF BREATH

Without the magic of *breath,* it is possible for a person to live anywhere between six and fifteen minutes; however, it is well to note that for every second past the *six-minute mark* the chances for complete recovery toboggan down-grade with devastating speed.

The need for the magic health secret of oxygen in the human body should be well known even to the most illiterate, but *how* it accomplishes the miracle of a long and rewarding life may need explaining. Oxygen destroys or eliminates *car-*

bon dioxide, a heavy, colorless, odorless gas. It is a waste product derived from cellular action within the body. It can only be fully removed by correct habits of breathing, and not always in the so-called *normal* function of breathing. Several times each day every man, woman and child should indulge at least a minute to a minute-and-a-half of *deep breathing.* This intake of fresh, pure air should be accomplished slowly and deliberately, taking care to retain each of the *breaths* at least *three seconds.*

Madeline S. was plagued with a heart condition that had compelled her to take early retirement. When she first registered for my class in better living she was not only *shaky,* but she seemed to be constantly on the verge of fainting. Acting on her doctor's advice, she carried small net-covered capsules in her purse to be used in an emergency. Obviously, she was in a bad way. For some unexplained reason none of my lectures seemed to ring a bell with Madeline until I described the magic in life-extending breath. The idea sounded so reasonable to her that she began a program of deep breathing that very day. In fact, she went about her new routine with so much enthusiasm that she came very close to fainting on the second day. "Too much oxygen all-at-once when you aren't used to it" was her doctor's verdict. "Cool it a little," he went on to say, "until your body can handle it." Following her doctor's advice she cut her breathing routine in half. From that point on, her recovery was truly magic. Today she is back on her job — a vibrant and exciting personality.

WHY FORCED BREATHING IS NEGATIVE

Forced, rapid breathing is almost without value. In fact, there is much evidence to support the contention of some authorities, — oxygen can only be absorbed and used by the body according *to need,* and definitely not in terms of a sudden excess supply.

REDUCE PHYSICAL ACTIVITY
FOR GREATEST BENEFITS

While it is true that many of the alleged dis-eases can be overcome by a regime of breathing exercises, it is well to note that the less physical activity that accompanies these movements, the greater will be the benefits *accruing* to the person using this magic key to long life. We fully realize that this statement is little short of heresy, but the facts are all-too-clear to be denied.

HOW CORRECT BREATHING
CAN ADD LIFE TO YOUR YEARS

The purpose of correct breathing is to prolong the happy enjoyment of life. To do this effectively requires that we cleanse the body of impurities several times each day. This does not mean that we should be intemperate in our pursuit of breath, nor that we indulge long periods of breathing *exercises,* but it does mean that we must satisfy body needs.

When I first met Martin J. he was quite plainly in a *run-down condition.* In fact, he was badly in need of both a mental and physical uplift. "What to do?" seemed to be written all over him. Years of dissipation had taken a heavy toll of his body energies to the point where he was dragging around "a still-warm corpse" — to hear him tell it. About two years earlier he had gone on a strictly vegetarian diet with the hope of regaining some of his lost health. His new life-style in nutrition had helped some, but something was missing. When he heard my lecture on the *Power of Breath,* he was *grasping at straws.* Reluctantly at first, he tried the three-second-breath routine. Gradually he increased the exercise until he was practicing deep breathing six times a day. Results were magic to him. Within a week he was not only feeling better, but he was also developing a new lease on life and he had gained three pounds. To him this was truly a miracle.

Because of Martin's intense new interest in better living, he was able to find a suitable selling job in a local health food store. Today he is the picture of vigorous health. His faith in deep breathing had renewed the spark of life in him. "To say that I am grateful for your suggestion," he told me, "would be a gross understatement."

THE MAGIC OF
CONSCIOUS BREATH

Now that we have made crystal clear the need for several periods of *real breathing* during each day, we are going to add the one most important magic advantage that can be gained from taking in fresh, pure air, above and beyond accepted practices of breathing.

With each breath be joyously conscious of the fact that you are also absorbing the magic of life-restoring energy.

Without any chance of equivocation, *breath* is our *main line* of contact with life itself. Since life was imparted to our bodies, we should always sustain this thrilling contact in a pleasurable state of mind. We can partake of this wonderful life-extending *force,* or leave it alone. The choice is up to you.

A DRAMATIC RECOVERY

One of the most remarkable stories ever to come to my attention was the dramatic recovery of the former Ice Capades star Janet Battista. She suffered from a loathsome affliction known as *varicose veins*. She told me what had happened to her. She had just received a contract to skate for the famous show when an exciting picnic holiday turned into a tragic accident for her — a smashup shattered both legs. She was compelled to enter the hospital where she remained for ten long months, barely tolerating a cumbersome cast.

When the cast was finally removed, Janet discovered, to her horror, that she had developed painful and unsightly vericose veins, an ailment completely unthinkable for a show girl. Naturally enough, her contract was tabled. Repeated trips to her doctor brought very little assurance. She was told that an operation was her only hope and even that had limitations. It was doubtful that her shapely legs would ever be restored to their "show time" appearance.

Undaunted by the verdict, Janet declared, bravely, that "There must be a natural way to heal these bloated veins." With not much more than sheer determination and an insatiable curiosity, she set about implementing a research program in which she delved into the secrets of every medical book available and every health book she could find that even closely touched upon her problem. She attended every better living lecture that was presented by the local university.

From all this searching, there gradually emerged a basic truth that could not be denied: Varicose veins could be healed once the basic cause had been isolated. The rest was easy. In her research, Janet had learned that impure blood was loaded with toxic wastes accumulating from (1) too little fresh water, (2) improper deep breathing, and (3) poor elimination.

Janet promptly set about a regime of deep breathing exercises that accomplished miracles in a few weeks. Before too long, her contract with Ice Capades was restored and she went back with the glamorous show for five happy and rewarding years.

HOW TO USE
THE MAGIC OF FRESH AIR
DURING SLEEP

I know that I am going to step on a lot of toes when I make this next assertion, but it is nonetheless true. Persons who insist upon sleeping with doors and windows tightly closed are just plain reckless. In addition to deliberately cutting off anywhere from ten to thirty years of good health, these misguided individuals are lessening vital mental and physical forces to the point where actual body deterioration sets in years ahead of time. The hours of sleep are supposed to be a time when the body can be restored, revitalized, and recharged with energy units. Without fresh air, this is impossible. It simply means that during the rest period your motor is still running but your generator has been slowed down to the point where the signal light is *red*. You are not replenishing energy units with this practice because vital life forces are not receiving the life-extending *charge*.

THE STRANGE SUPERSTITION
ABOUT NIGHT AIR

For many years people have closed their windows against the supposed bad effects of night air. The origin of this superstitious idea of closed windows is lost in history, but its ill effects are still with us today. Alert persons, mindful of steadily improving attitudes toward this question, are aware that so-called sinus irritations, the common cold and other respiratory ailments can usually be traced to a *lack* of fresh air at night, rather than too much. Queer ideas of diet and off-beat habits of living are more likely to be the villains.

Should you be one of the persons fearful of the *bugaboos* of the night, just try coming into the twentieth century for awhile — you might like it, and most important, you might be able to latch on to twenty-five or thirty more years of happy, enjoyable living.

In the event that you are still not convinced of the value of breathing *fresh air,* let us regard for a moment the basic facts of physiology, all of which serve to sustain my beliefs. In all ordinary breathing, a person will inhale and exhale approximately *one pint* of air with each breath. In the study of body processes, this is described as the *tidal breath,* the natural minimum ebb-and-flow of air necessary to sustain life. This level of breathing is the lowest possible *common denominator* in the living sequence. It simply maintains the pattern of existence. It does not recharge the human reserves of electric energy.

HOW TO USE
YOUR "VITAL CAPACITY"

It is known that at the deepest possible inhalation of breath the lungs of most persons will hold about four quarts of air. This is described as *vital capacity.* When we reach this point of inspiration, we are making contact with the vast, free-flowing electric current of the Universe. We are recharging our basic life forces. With each of these deep breaths we absorb life-giving and life-extending energies. We reduce the expenditure of our vital electric potential to a minimum. With each deep inhalation we approach the ideal in attaining or exceeding *maintenance* breathing. This is for the purpose of achieving the goal of a long and happy life, right up to the point where the normal *friction* of daily existence makes it impossible to further lessen the outflow of our *electric reserves*.

In the act of recharging, or revitalizing the life forces with deep inhalations of fresh air, it is essential that the lungs first be emptied of all *stale air*. To do this effectively, simply *exhale* until it is impossible to release any more air, then begin to gulp in air, not noisily, or obviously, for the very plain reason that you might want to take your inhalations while in public, and it isn't necessary to make observers think you are off your rocker, or about ready to collapse. With each big gulp, increase the intake each time until you have reached the point where it is impossible to inhale more. At this point hold the breath for *three seconds* only. Repeat this performance two or three times, but cautiously in the beginning. Too much ozygen will cause you to become dizzy. Remember, the body can accept just so much of an electric charge at a time, and no more. It is far better to repeat the inhalation every hour or so during the day, and far more beneficial.

HOW YOU CAN ACTIVATE
YOUR RESTORATIVE DYNAMIC

Some few enlightened educators across the nation are beginning to realize the full value of correct breathing, with a steadily growing number of them taking steps to introduce *breathing spells* within the established academic programs.

Fortunately, this forward movement is gaining acceptance from all levels of scholastic activity, from the elementary groups right on through the post graduate centers of learning in law, medicine and technology.

With several semesters of limited, often casual experiments in this field, results are already beginning to pile up an impressive array of favorable evidence. The heretofore disinterested or inadequate student gradually becomes fired with renewed enthusiasm for his study assignments. This situation has been strikingly apparent among grammar school children, often the most susceptible to such training, but even more imposing are the results reported from college and post graduate *researchers*.

Mary K., a retired elementary school teacher, was a regular member of my class in better living. One day she decided to enter the University with the avowed purpose of winning her doctorate in education — not that she needed the additional credits, but for the sheer joy of accomplishment. Much to her chagrin, she discovered it was tough going — not only to keep up with the young professor in taking required notes, but to stay alert enough to absorb the knowledge she should learn. When she heard my lecture on the "Power of Breath," she decided to give the deep breathing routine a good workout. Within three days improvement was so noticeable that it attracted the professor's attention — and within the following two weeks she was able to add materially to the class discussions because of her thirty years' experience as a classroom teacher.

From then on, Mary was like a person "reborn." Examinations were a breeze, and when her final disseration was nearing the deadline she was able to complete the prodigious task on schedule and in top form. When it came time to don her mortarboard and colorfully-lined graduating gown to receive her coveted award, she was named the outstanding candidate of her class — and all of this happened on her seventieth birthday.

That *breath* and *life* are synonymous all dictionaries agree. Breath *is* life. Still, how few there are who give this subject serious thought, or even consider for a moment the idea of including study of *breath* as a means of extending the life cycle, or worse, make any attempt to discover the basic movements so essential for revitalizing or restoring needed body energies.

Your breathing capacity may be only average and your mental and physical ailments may be many — or at least complicated. In that case you must remember, especially in the beginning, that it will be extremely important for you to pay more attention to your breathing habits. Try going through the regular three-second breathing movement several times each day (as presented within this book for your use). Correct breathing is a vital part of my philosophy of life-extension, and as such I consider it an essential means of attaining an active, fully creative, and vigorous life expression.

THE MAGIC POWER
OF INTERNAL CLEANSING

The study of *right breathing* discloses many interesting and many surprising facts which can, when used according to natural law, greatly aid a serious reader in either preventing, arresting, or conquering many so-called dis-eases. A clean mind and a *breath-cleansed* body will not admit a malfunction of any kind, but even here nature has its laws of correspondence which must forever remain inviolate, for the author of cosmic laws is Intelligence itself, therefore the improvement of our breathing habits is essentially a part of our present concern.

To expect nature to serve us and to accept the treasures of health, well being, and a long and creative life that she has in store for us, we must also be greatly desirous of regenerating our physical body. Man, in seeking the revitalization of his electric energies, must ever remember that two great factors are at work, helping him at all times toward his goal of rejuvenation. These are: *Crystallization* and *focalization*. Without the union of both, polarity of his electric forces is impossible. In this day of overly-rated *sophistication*, this might sound like something *way-out*, but one day it will be regarded as just plain common sense.

THE ENERGIZED "SPARK OF LIFE"

One should never forget for a single minute that it is *breath* that upholds and sustains life, for what is breath but *agitation, motion, continuity of operation* — the antithesis or exact opposite of stagnation and decay.

The free flow of *breath* coming into the lungs touches the inner body with a new spark of life. Breath is organized operation, organized agitation. Air is the surrounding part of the elements we use to complete the function of breathing. *All life-creating energy lies within the breath.*

To the extent that we pay attention to our breath and breathing, we will realize more and more through consideration and thoughtfulness, the power contained within this form of agitation known as breath and breathing. As we grow in knowledge of this bodily function, we are thus enabled to retain all of the elements within the province of the *dynamics,* ordinarily called lungs with their several bellows or wings.

We are now ready to review our breathing exercise with the definite object in view of establishing a base for all of the keys to the magic of long life — with the ever present aim of organizing our use of these several methods into a practical, easily used program. One that we can apply at convenient times as we go about our normal everyday activities.

YOUR INDIVIDUAL BREATH —
A RESERVOIR OF POWER

As we have previously mentioned, our FIRST STEP to all of our breathing movements should be the PRELUDE BREATH. This can best be accomplished in the following manner:

(1) Begin by breathing short breaths. One breath in, one breath out. In, out — in, out — six or more times.

(2) After the sixth or seventh time, completely *empty* the lungs with a long OUT. You will then be fully prepared to *inhale* a deep, full breath and retain this intake for no more than three seconds. You can safely repeat this exercise two or three times.

In the event that you are using the breath for therapeutic purposes, after consulting your doctor, it is normally safe to go through the breathing movements every hour during the day.

Science has proved beyond any doubt that food takes on bright new dimensions when correct breathing habits are established. You will learn why when you begin to use the next step toward the magic of a long and happy life.

THOUGHTS ABOUT
THE SEVENTH MAGIC SECRET

(1) Breath is our ever-present contact with our vital life forces. Never forget for one moment that breath and life are synonymous. Breath is in fact *life*.

(2) Each person can absorb and *use* the intake of energies that can be derived from three to five periods of deep breathing every day, providing the exercises do not extend over *ninety seconds.*

(3) The physical body needs to be cleansed of impurities several times each day. Deep breathing is one of the essential practices that must be included in the daily routines. In addition to the benefit of cleansing, an even greater advantage will be gained in the renewal of body energies.

(4) Before indulging in a *deep breathing exercise,* the lungs should be completely emptied of all *stale air.*

(5) Many dis-eases and physical upsets simply disappear when a daily regime of deep breathing is made a part of our pattern of living.

10

THE EIGHTH
MAGIC HEALTH SECRET:
HOW TO USE
THE RESTORATIVE POWER
OF STRETCHING AND TENSING

A happy routine of stretching and tensing can extend your life span many years. Countless research projects have revealed again and again that a top physical condition is not dependent upon how much exercise a person indulges — either in tedious regimes of calisthenics, sports or other body actions — but rather upon certain movements that are described as stretching and tensing all body muscles in order to maintain bodily strength and vitality.

One of the greatest distortions of fact prevailing in the world today is the claim that *physical fitness* demands rugged exercise. Fifty-mile hikes, participation sports, annual hunting expeditions, or unusual *yard work sprees* are but symptoms of this great urge of the human family to *overdo*.

Where and when these intemperate indulgences originated is lost in the dim mists of history, but more than likely when man first began to emerge into *consciousness*, a natural vanity prodded him on to show his prowess, and the quest for leadership was on in full force.

DANGER IN STRENUOUS EXERCISE

Too much exercise can reduce your chances of long life. During the tens-of-thousands of years that have elapsed since Man, the human *expression*, first realized his *expanding* potential, the needs and urgencies of survival have changed. The compulsions of these early days still linger with us, however, even though the necessity for these *binges* of physical activity have long since passed.

Actually, two, or possibly five minutes of *resistance*, or tensing of all of the body muscles is all that is required in order to keep any man, woman or child in top physical condition. The aim, the intent, and the purpose of our endeavors should be to delay physical maturity. This cannot be done by strenuous programs of exercises, early morning runs, or 36 holes of golf. In truth, any of these greatly over-rated practices can drain off essential body energies so fast that the miracle of long life can be reduced as much as *forty to sixty percent*.

A NEW CONCEPT

Through the years there has emerged a new concept in the area of developing and maintaining good health and physi-

cal vigor. Within this frame of reference, two outstanding programs stand out preeminently. Number one in this category is
the ancient and highly revered system known as *Yoga.*

I first learned about Yoga during a delightful and revealing luncheon meeting with the late Paramhansa Yogananda,
spiritual leader of the Self Realization Fellowship.

In response to my question, "Is Yoga strictly for spiritual
development?" his emphatic answer was, "No!" Then he went
on to explain, "It is our hope that persons who enroll in our
Yoga classes at the Los Angeles Temple will be so impressed by
the effectiveness of the program on a purely physical level that
they will have a quickened curiosity about aspects of Yoga that
are spiritual.

"By practicing the postures of Yoga," Yogananda went on,
"It is possible to experience the bodily disciplines that afford
physical health."

Later on in our interview, Yogananda went on to comment,
"Those ancient people of India, knew what modern medical
scientists discovered only recently — that the body and mind
constantly interact."

Shortly after this interview, I was privileged to attend one
of the class sessions. I was greatly impressed with the almost
worshipful attitude of the group. At the close of the class meeting, I had the opportunity to speak with a man whom I shall
call Don, a pleasant man of middle age. "When I joined the
class, I had just about everything wrong with my mental and
physical well being. Now I am a greatly renewed person. I
honestly believe I have added many enjoyable years to my life
span."

The other program that presently seems to be attracting
nation wide attention is the system known as *Isometric Tension,*
or, as the originator of the routine, Donald J. Salls, Ed.D.,
describes it: "almost effortless exercise."

The plan was created by Dr. Salls when he helped to coach
the world famous winning football team known as the "Crim-
son Tide," players whose achievements are now legendary.

Copies of the chart describing the ten static exercises can be obtained by writing to the Salls Foundation, Anniston, Alabama. However, there is one word of caution: you had better consult your doctor and follow his advice to the letter before you begin the program.

WHY YOU SHOULD ABANDON COMPETITIVE SPORTS

When the truth emerges from the vast research projects now under way, I predict that all present school athletic programs will be abandoned; all amateur athletic contests will become relics of our historic past; and all weekend sports enthusiasts will find relaxation and gain needed strength from nothing more strenuous than walking woodland trails, or indulging in a brief, leisurely swim.

In time, the only person who will engage in the rugged, often boisterous, always questionable *participation* sports, will be the professional player who is willing to trade his life-sustaining energies for the transient and doubtful rewards of cash and a moment of glory.

SELECTING YOUR OWN PROGRAM OF DIRECTED MOVEMENT

As we jet-propel ourselves into the age of atoms, automation and abbreviated bikinis, with an ever-growing tendency to embrace a worthy study of beauty in art, nature and philosophy, more and more enlightened persons will discover that the very peak of physical well-being can be attained and perpetuated by a daily program of stretching and tensing body muscles that does not at any time exceed five minutes.

When we attempt to isolate and bring into clear focus exactly what is meant by the type of body movements required for perfect physical conditioning, we will start with a simple premise.

Here's all you have to do. Just make sure you regularly move your body and limbs, and gently resist these pushing, pulling or bending motions. In other words, stretch your body and tense your muscles each day. Any natural movement of the arms, legs, or torso in which a push, pull or bend is resisted gently, will eventually bring any person as close to physical maturity as he should ever be — short of the maximum of seventy-five or eighty years. After that the magic of long life is yours.

WHY YOUR ATTITUDE TOWARD EXERCISE
SHOULD APPROACH THE AGE OF REASON

You won't find this idea popular with any of the colorfully advertised and heavily promoted exercise parlors, or muscle-building courses, but the truth of the matter is that we are now approaching the age of reason in our physical fitness programs. Before too long, intelligent men and women the nation over will come to realize the fallacy of working up a big sweat in order to maintain good health.

Somewhere deep in the shadowy beginnings of mankind some contemplative person decided that all of the rough-and-tumble body movements common to his era of living were just too tedious. With this unpretentious curtain raiser for the new age, time marched on for thousands of years while scattered groups managed to toss the idea around until widely dispersed remnants of these various movements began to collect and use the teachings of the early Zend-Avesta peoples. This particular ethnic group is commonly believed to come from the foothills of the Himalayas. However, all that we are concerned with here is the origin of an idea that took so long to filter into the consciousness of mankind.

At the present time all of the Communist nations are using the theory of *isometric tension,* a term applied to this form of exercise by the noted football coach, Dr. Donald J. Salls, to the consternation of overly zealous athletes and the persons who direct their strongly competitive activities.

HOW YOU CAN SELECT YOUR OWN STRETCHING AND TENSING PROGRAM

There are many systems, courses of study — and naturally enough, exponents for pay — of the art of *tensing* muscles for the purpose of *creating* good health and well being. These range all the way from the poetic and colorfully named T'ai Chi exercise to the practical and simplified body movements originated by Dr. Salls. This latter group of limited exercise is my favorite for the reason that it is a "daily program of almost *motionless* exercises, designed to provide physical fitness without strenuous effort."

WHY MODERATION IS YOUR ANSWER

However, it is equally essential to note that over-stretching, tensing or exertion will tend to dissipate body energies for no good purpose. Even the over-use of brain cells will wear away the vital electric forces of *being* unless there is a *rhythm* in one's endeavor. For example, long tedious hours of study or application to the solving of a stubborn problem must be lightened with a leisure break, or time out for a good *breather* in which the three-second-breath is indulged at least twice, followed by fully five minutes of relaxation, during which time the mind is allowed to relax completely.

THERE IS NO ROOM
FOR DISAGREEMENT

At the present time there are many research projects active in this field. It is only natural that with so many points of view brought to bear on the subject, a vast amount of disagreement will follow each of the summations, influenced of course by a tendency on the part of the researchers to work *on the bias*. This will be hotly denied as being contrary to the purpose of probing for truth, but nonetheless I have seen it happen too many times for this reality to be evaded.

Again and again, research has proved that the *right kind* of body movements is far more valuable *and lasting* than the extent of indulgence in physical training programs of any description. There is an overwhelming array of evidence accumulating to support the principle of *isometric* tension as described by Dr. Salls, rather than strenuous athletic programs.

All college and high-school competitive games, gymnastics, and spectator sports are promoted for only two reasons:

(1) to keep under control, by draining off, the exhuberant and life-sustaining energies of young people and

(2) to make money.

It is all that simple.

ATHLETICS AND MATURITY

As people become more concerned with achieving true maturity, the emphasis on strenuous sports will fade away. As parents and teachers come to realize the need to develop the bodies of children slowly and carefully, competitive games will be taught less and less.

I declare emphatically that the more healthful way is to give proper attention to the maturity concept. With this idea in practice, there would soon be a much lower percentage of high school graduates interested only in play. There would be a much higher percentage of high school graduates interested in furthering their work skills, and in developing more social responsibility as well.

More concern should be expressed and shared by parents, teachers, and other educators for the physical welfare of the child. It is impossible to develop a well-balanced mind in a poorly-balanced, over-exercised body. It is equally impossible to develop the factors that are needed for a long and happy life in a physical body that has been drained of its vital energies by over-exertion and under-nutrition. To gain the benefits of a greatly extended life span, *balance* in the life process should be achieved before the age of fourteen.

Because most of us regard the day-after-day *repetition* of tedious exercises to be quite a bore — completely without stimulus or imagination — the idea of devoting a few brief moments every day to the process of recharging, revitalizing and energizing the body, should have great appeal, especially when the rewards are so great. Life will then take on a whole new world of meaning when the full *active ingredients* of food, breath, sex, mind, rhythm, vibration and tensing and stretching are used only to the limits of their regenerative potential.

THOUGHTS ABOUT
THE EIGHTH SECRET

(1) We should use great restraint in matters of exercise in order to *delay* physical maturity as long as possible.

(2) No person who is sincerely interested in attaining the magic of long life will indulge more than a few minutes of tensing, stretching or *resistance* exercises every day.

(3) The idea of tensing, or isometric tension as it is now called, is not new. The practice originated with the Zend-Avesta peoples thousands of years ago.

(4) The benefits that can be achieved with a few brief moments of *tensing* each day are without limit *and the years of life that can be added unto each individual are priceless.*

(5) Fifty-mile hikes, rugged participation sports and unusual work sprees are extravagantly wasteful of body energies.

11

THE NINTH MAGIC SECRET: THE DYNAMIC PRINCIPLE OF VIBRATION

You can influence your own bodily health by applying the dynamic force of vibration, a revitalizing, strengthening force of nature you can use to restore yourself and increase your life span. Making use of vibration requires no mechanical aids of any kind, but I will explain how inexpensive mechanical devices can help this powerful process.

As you know, *vibration* is a fundamental action in nature. Without vibration there would be no life. With this pulsation of energy that expands and contracts rhythmically, all life ebbs and flows. So many patterns of life proceed in patterns of vibration that study of these patterns enables scientists to know and predict many behaviors of man and other creatures of the earth. It is a pulsation that seems to emanate from one central source in the universe.

THE REGENERATIVE
SECRETS OF NATURE

Early in the twentieth century bold men of science began to probe these *unknowns* with astonishing results. By 1926, Sir J. C. Bose had managed to construct an extremely sensitive contraption with which he was able to detect the *rhythmical electrical* changes in the stems of plants. From these early explorations into the secrets of the Universe, there were myriad forays made into the vast unknown habits of nature, but it remained for the renowned researcher, Dr. Frank Brown of Northwestern University, to come up with a postulate that the source of these *directions,* or instructions, comes from *some outside source.* Several possibilities are suggested, but the one that seems to fit known truths with the greatest accuracy is *cosmic radiation.*

HOW YOU CAN NOW CONTACT
THIS NATURAL HEALING POWER

Because we know the genesis of being, the next logical step is to learn *when* and *how* to make contact with *and absorb* a fair share of this revitalizing force for the purpose of restoring the energies of the physical body. It is well to point out that all of the secrets you are learning must be used in order to attain the perfect result — the magic of a long and happy life.

Shortly after the close of World War II, the mechanical version of vibrating tables, chairs, pads and hand-vibrators burst upon the American scene with almost boom proportions. At the close of this chapter we will explore the idea more fully.

One enterprise that fascinated me greatly was the vibrating bed. After a long day of travel or a particularly heavy lecture schedule during the day and evening, I always tried to locate a motel or hotel with beds that featured the restoring qualities of vibration. When I could find one that could be regulated from "strong" to a mild "purr," I was especially delighted.

Normally, the charge for fifteen minutes of relaxing comfort was twenty-five cents. With such a small investment I was able to unwind completely in a matter of minutes. Most of the time I was sound asleep before my alloted time ran out, no matter how uptight the affairs of the day had made me.

Another example that came to light shortly after the advent of hand-vibrators was reported to me by Clark S., a barber in Colorado. It seems that Clark was faced with early retirement because an arthritic condition in his hands was rapidly becoming so painful that continuing his trade was more than he could bear.

One day when he was on the verge of giving up, an enterprising barber supply salesman introduced him to one of the better hand type appliances to be used on the back and neck of customers. During the few moments of the demonstration, Clark's hands were so greatly relieved of pain that he bought one on the spot. Thereafter, every chance he got during the day he massaged his hands vigorously with his new-found *therapy*. Almost within hours of each application, his pain lessened and within two weeks of this procedure his hands were so much improved that he gave up all thought of retiring.

ASSIMILATING THIS DYNAMIC ENERGY

In order to receive *and assimilate* the cosmic radiations of life, it is essential that the person wanting to accept a new supply of *energy units* do so in consciousness and at a high level of vibrational build-up. To the uninitiated this might sound like so much *gobbledegook,* but actually the feeling is known to every living person; it is easily generated, almost at will, and this feeling of great elation can be maintained for several seconds at a time.

To accomplish this highly receptive period of revitalization, all you need to do is isolate yourself in a quiet, secluded place where complete relaxation is possible. You must remain in this place for some time. This restorative period is often mistakenly described as meditation.

When your physical body is completely at ease, begin the vibrational build-up by clearing the mind of all trivia. This can be done very simply by repeating the words: *power, strength, love, beauty, color, music, flowers,* and so on — any word that seems to excite a pleasurable feeling. Within moments you will be conscious of a vitalizing glow that will permeate your whole body. When this feeling of super-elation is at its height, you will be in full contact with the ultimate source of all life-giving energy. During this period of great elation, or receptivity, the life forces of your body will be recharged, energized and vitalized. A glow of supreme exultation will flood every nerve and fiber of your being. You will be greatly renewed in spirit.

HOW YOU CAN ACHIEVE
A HIGHLY ENERGIZED
VIBRATIONAL BUILD-UP WITH WORDS

Say, for example, that each word has a vibrational build-up factor of *five.* With *twenty* power-packed words you can raise your vibrational level to 100% within a very few minutes. With this revved-up natural source of dynamic energy going for you, you can heal, restore, or extend your span of happy, active years almost at will and accomplish or overcome nearly all obstacles.

HERE IS YOUR ENERGIZED WORD LIST

(1)	Power	(11)	Glow
(2)	Strength	(12)	Drive
(3)	Vigor	(13)	Sparkling
(4)	Energy	(14)	Bold
(5)	Force	(15)	Ecstasy
(6)	Mighty	(16)	Pleasure
(7)	Strong	(17)	Joy
(8)	Vitality	(18)	Charm
(9)	Health	(19)	Thrilling
(10)	Spirit	(20)	LOVE

ARE YOU READY FOR THIS MIRACLE OF REGENERATION?

To the novice, the use of this particular step can be very *powerful stuff*. It should not be indulged too often, especially in the beginning. With continued practice, the qualities of assimilation can be improved to the point where the exercise can be used as much as three or four times each day, unless, of course, a person is confronted with a period of illness or great stress. The only point to bear in mind is that too much can be disturbing, just as too little can be costly in badly needed units of energy. In the process of *recharging,* it is well to remember that it is virtually impossible to reduce the daily expenditure of energy to zero. Should this point be reached and sustained, it is quite obvious that the life span could be extended indefinitely.

THE ENERGIZING POWERS
OF A VIBRATIONAL BUILD-UP

Medical Science has established the fact that a *node,* or a slightly raised point of highly specialized muscle and nerve tissue situated in the wall of the upper chamber of the heart, is activated by the basic body energies, and just prior to each *beat,* manages to discharge a minute amount of *electric current,* thus causing the heart to function within the area of its life-sustaining purpose. But up until recently no one had created an instrument capable of measuring the strength of the energy units remaining in the body reservoir of life forces.

It is now known that when the "storage battery" of electrical energies that sustain life have been worn down, it is possible to *recharge* or rebuild these vital powers that have been depleted by questionable habits of living, breathing and thinking.

How this can be achieved has been revealed to you in a carefully planned, *step-by-step* program. This outline of procedures is basic and factual. Only once do we approach the threshold of the unknown, but only to parallel the great mass of investigation and study that is now going on in universities and research centers. For this reason we now undertake the examination of the one ponderable with which we are confronted in the probe of the several secrets of vibrant confident living.

In order to placate the *doubting Thomases* of the world whose hardened mental apparatus is not susceptible to new *wrinkles,* we will assume for the time being that this is the *cause* of all that we know as life, and the unlimited supplier of *life-giving energies.* I assert with great emphasis that vibration, or *cosmic radiation* is the source — and one of the few remaining secrets leading to a rewarding life expression.

HOW YOU CAN USE
THE FOUR SOURCES
OF ENERGIZED VIBRATION

Within this study we are concerned with the basic *cause* of vibrations that recharge, regenerate and restore *energy units* that serve to extend and *expand* the life principle. We have explored at some length the most powerful of these forces, now we will examine the remaining four contributing or supporting origins of life-giving energies.

LIGHT. All of us are familiar with the term and condition that we describe as *light,* but all too few of us are fully aware of the fact that light is, and a cause of, *vibration.* This *wave of energy* coming from out of space can extend or destroy life. Our aim now is to reveal how you can make the greatest possible use of light for the purpose of revitalizing your life forces.

What I am about to say will shock some faddists, anger many devotees of *sun bathing,* and bring bitter protest from the younger *muscle beach crowd*, but the facts are unmistakable. *The sun can shorten your life span just as easily as it can extend it.*

For the purpose of prolonging life, no person should expose himself to sunlight "in the raw" for more than seven minutes at a time. To achieve the greatest good from exposure to the sun, the body should be without covering of any kind. Some individuals can take seven minutes each front and back without any ill effects, but anything more tends to reverse the process of extending the life span.

Admittedly, there is some argument over whether the morning or afternoon sunlight is better for the purpose of recreating energies. For myself, I have solved the problem in this manner: I know that under all ordinary circumstances that I exhaust one full unit of energy within about five hours after rising in the morning; therefore, I prefer to take my five to seven minutes, both front and back, near the noon hour. When I can do this I am able to regenerate my body forces at a time when ever nerve and cell is most receptive to the revitalizing energies of the *Universal Light*. Should the day be cloudy, there are sun lamps that do the job almost as effectively. There is a valid natural reason for alternate periods of darkness and light; however, it is only pertinent here for us to note that it must be observed.

There is one point of caution that perhaps should be injected at this time—in the event that you are *thin-skinned*, or especially sensitive to sunlight, it might be better to cover the body with a thin coating of vegetable oil. I know this is *messy*, because I have to do it this way, but it does pay off. A quick warm shower afterward *without soap* will remove most of the oil, leaving your skin feeling soft and velvety.

Mary B., at age 45, was aging fast. Her skin was rapidly becoming dry, wrinkled and leathery. Creams, lotions and beauty oils were serving no good purpose. She had been an avid sun-bather since her early teens. Now she was paying the price—and at a time of life when she most wanted to be attractive. She had devoted herself to the "good life" as a career woman and now the "fiddler" demanded payment. When Mary first joined my class in Better Living, she looked at least sixty. At first she was inclined to give me an argument about sun bathing, but finally she cut the practice from her daily routine. With a generous use of rich oils from head to toe she was soon regaining her youthful appearance. Her hair began to take on the luster of youth—and of great importance to her, body aches and pains began to disappear and a new zest for life was flowing through her otherwise well-formed body—so much so that before the second semester was over she attracted the attention of a rugged bachelor who had been caught up in the maelstrom of war and never married. In the morning's mail recently I received a cheery note from Mary in which she said, "I'm getting married this coming Saturday and I would very much like to have you 'give the bride away'—all because of what you have done for me."

SOUND. The beneficial effects of harmonized sound waves, or *vibrations*, and the disturbing, often harmful consequences of just plain *noise*, is too well known to explore at this point. "Rock-and-Roll" music, for example, is completely demoralizing and degenerative. Suffice to say that a very practical reason—the *recreation of energy*—is reason enough to justify the great popularity of soft music being *piped* in to work areas, shopping centers and restaurants. Even cows respond by giving more milk—and hens are stimulated to lay more eggs when soft music is played.

In this connection, it is well to emphasize that persons or animals subjected to long periods of even the most delightful music, do not benefit as much as groups that enjoy intervals of pleasant *restful silence*. Even the most harmonized of sound combinations finally reach a point of *diminishing returns*, and this includes long-drawn-out symphonies, operas and concerts. All that these impressive musical presentations offer the individual is another form of a cultural *binge*.

For the purposes of sustaining or *regenerating* body energies, a good recording of a favorite symphony *played only at widely* spaced intervals during the day, has far greater value.

When I first knew Annie R., she was a lively, pert, vivacious young woman in her middle twenties. She was under no pressure to seek a career. However, she began to realize that she had too much leisure time on her hands. Raucous and loud music was sweeping the land with its primitive beat and Annie was caught up in the aboriginal craze—so much so that she was neglecting herself in order to take part in the primal binges. She was rapidly becoming a nervous wreck. She admitted she had tried marijuana to steady her nerves. When she first attended one of my public lectures, she was so uptight she couldn't sit through one of my hour-long presentations. Three times during my talk she had to slip out of the room for a few drags on a cigarette. At the close of a discussion of the topic of sound, she rather timidly approached me with the question: "What does a person do who has gone bananas over loud music?"

Suspecting this might be a trick question, I countered with one of my own: "Do you like being the way you are now?" "No" was her emphatic response. "In that case," I replied, "stop listening to the barbaric stuff as of right now." A look of shocked surprise spread over her face at so simple a solution. "I'll try" was her parting shot.

Apparently, Annie really did "try"—because improvement was noticeable almost immediately. By the end of the semester she was behaving quite normally. When my class opened again in the fall, she was right there in the front row—obviously well along toward becoming a normal human being.

COLOR. It would be difficult to imagine a world without color. Basically, color is simply vibration. The colors that we identify as red, blue or yellow, are nothing more than varying wave lengths of light. In fact, color is one of the properties of light, just as a pitch or tone is one of the properties of sound.

Within this brief study, it is our aim to show how color, in connection with cosmic radiation, light, sound and mechanical vibration, can be used to recharge the physical body with badly needed supplies of electric energy. It might seem a little weird, especially in the beginning, should you picture an attempt to use all of the revitalizing factors at one time. But it can be done, and very successfully, although I wouldn't recommend it for a starting exercise. The result could very easily *vibrate* you right into a complete tizzy. Obviously, this practice is extremely potent and should be indulged with great caution as you initiate your program of *regeneration*.

The problem of how to select the color, or colors, most beneficial to each individual is important. *Red* is physical; *yellow* is intellectual; and *blue* is spiritual. Each person has a basic color. Your color can be any one of the three primaries, or a combination of them. In the event that you do not know your *principle*, or sustaining inclinations, you will, of necessity, have to depend upon your intuition, or *responses* to color in order to determine the one most likely to be helpful.

It is quite essential that once you know your basic color, you should immediately take steps to surround yourself with varying shades of this particular interpretation of light. While it is true that each of the secrets you are now learning contributes only a small portion of the needed sustaining, or regenerating energies, it is nonetheless important that each factor must be used to the full extent of its potential in order to achieve the ultimate goal of joyous, confident living. The one significant quality of color is that once it is accomplished, little time is involved in deriving benefits from this vibration.

Should you entertain any doubt about the advantages of the vibrations of either light, color, or sound, just try to imagine what it would be like to even exist without light—to live in a room, or work in an area with a predominant color that was even slightly offensive—or listen to a sound that seemed to claw at every nerve and fiber of your being.

Mabel M. tells an exciting story of how she turned from a dull housewifely type into a radiant personality simply by changing colors—not only in her dress preferences, but in all of the rooms of her home. Being an avid reader of home and family type magazines, she was exposed to some outlandish color combinations in painting and decorating for family living quarters. Before long it was obvious that the freakish mixture she had achieved was not only disturbing to her husband, but it had the children at each other's throats much of the time. Quite by accident, she happened to sit in on my lecture about vibration. When I mentioned the effects color could have on a person's life, she nearly jumped out of her chair. After the lecture she waited for me at the door.

Without preamble, she asked, "What do you say is my basic color?" Looking her over carefully I answered, "Offhand I would say you are a spiritual type—and blue is the right color for you." "Good grief!" was her response. "I can't always dress in blue or paint the house and all the rooms in blue." "No," I answered, "but you can use any soft variable shade of blue or green and probably achieve the result you want."

Months passed with no further word from Mabel—until one day while I was giving a repeat of my lecture on vibration, she appeared—a trim and glowing person. Her opening remark was most revealing: "You will never know what your talk did for me, but I do want you to know that I am very grateful"— and as she turned away, she displayed a great big smile of genuine appreciation.

MECHANICAL VIBRATION. Now we come to the one *vibration* that still is a matter of some controversy. This is true, in spite of the fact that millions of hand-vibrators are now in use and, during the past twenty-five years many companies have entered into the business of manufacturing vibrating chairs, vibrating tables, and even spot vibrators for the feet, back, or shoulders. Some motels have installed vibrating beds for the purpose of inducing a restful night's sleep.

Regardless of how you feel about the matter, too much evidence has piled up in favor of *mechanical vibration* to dismiss lightly this vital aid to a glowing life expression.

However, there is one quite important point to consider. There are about as many vibrations of vibrational strength as there are tones in the scale of sound. These run the gamut from a mere purr, to a veritable jack-hammer-type of shaking that is of little value—perhaps even harmful. Obviously, each person responds better to his or her own level of vibration. The only way that this can be determined is to try out various pieces of equipment until one is found that delivers the flow of vibration that is most rewarding for you. Better yet, find one that can be adjusted to body needs.

For those who find great benefit from sleeping in a vibrating bed, it is quite plain that the very mild, or purr type is to be favored.

Now we come to the part that might seem *weird* to the beginner of our vibrational studies that was mentioned some time back. Whenever it is possible, I like to stretch out *raw*, on a cool, clean sheet over a mildly vibrating bed, under a blue sky at high noon. With soft strains of a recorded music barely perceptible, I can attain a vibrational build-up equal to the highest values of life-sustaining cosmic radiation and thus receive the full flow of healing energies, creative powers and perceptive qualities that can be bestowed upon me by nature.

When you activate all of the magic secrets of long life, you will unlock a vast new treasure chest of knowledge about you as an individual. Science is just now beginning to penetrate the secrets of nature—little known mysteries that possess unusual life-sustaining powers. For example, just now emerging is the concept of using ultra-sound in healing, in surgery and for the relief of pain.

AN ESCAPE FROM
THE RAVAGES OF ARTHRITIS

Jack R. indirectly found relief from a very painful arthritic condition in both hands with a vibrating pad. For some time it was getting to be almost unbearable when he tried to pick up a paper and worse whenever he tried to pick up any heavy object. One day a throw rug slipped out from under him with the result that he suffered an extremely painful hip injury. Liniments, massages and hot sitz baths offered little relief.

During one of his visits to the doctor, it was suggested that a vibrating pad might help. Jack R. was skeptical but figured anything was worth a try. It took some doing for him to find the pad he wanted, but finally he located one in a thrift shop. Dutifully, he applied the strongly-vibrating pad to both hips night and morning until the pain slowly disappeared. Nature might have taken care of the situation anyway, but the most amazing result was now in evidence. Because he had to hold the vibrating pad on his hips with his hands he had achieved a miracle. The pain and stiffness in his *hands* was also gone completely!

When Jack related his story in class I was really surprised to learn how many persons had a vibrating contraption of some kind in their homes and had only used them indifferently for their aches and pains. From that day on, happy reports of good results poured into our group meetings with almost every session.

CAN ULTRA-SOUND
BE CLASSED AS VIBRATION?

For more than half a century an extension of vibration known as *ultra-sound* has been both praised and condemned.

When the idea first came to my attention one form of the therapy was known as diathermy. Unfortunately, the poorly considered propaganda for diathermy prevented consideration of any merit the device might possess. Now that a new concept has exploded upon the American scene, proponents of the use of ultra-sound are too prestigious to brush off lightly. For example, Richard N. Steigerwalt, chief physical therapist at the Allentown, Pennsylvania Sacred Heart Hospital, reports fantastic results with ultra-sound. In the hands of a competent doctor it is known that the relative intensity of the ultra-sound waves is of crucial importance.

It is generally conceded that sound can destroy or heal. In the hands of a novice, sound-therapy could be a disaster. However, when used at proper intensities and frequencies there is a strong possibility that it might be effective in treating all forms of aches and pains.

Admittedly, sound wave therapy is not a miracle, but according to recognized authorities, including James E. Griffin, Ph.D., who had studied the concept extensively, the new technique has considerable merit. It should be investigated with a completely open mind.

THOUGHTS ABOUT
THE NINTH MAGIC SECRET

(1) You can improve your health with vibration, a powerful force of cosmic radiation.

(2) Sunlight, one of the carriers of cosmic radiation, is healthful for you, but you should limit your exposure to this powerful, life-giving medium to seven-minute sunbathing periods—front and back.

(3) When used properly, sound waves can be a powerful vibration for health.

(4) Color, one of the properties of light, has healing powers.

(5) You will find mechanical vibrations a helpful form of artificial stimulation for your body. These vibrations can be safely supplied by a number of devices available in today's market, from little hand-vibrators to expensive vibrating tables. You can only determine which device you would use from your own experience.

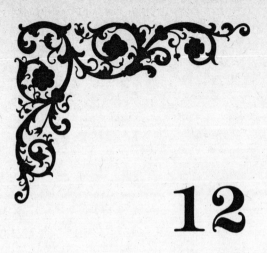

12

HOW ONE MAN LEARNED
TO USE
THE MAGIC SECRETS
OF LONG LIFE

It has often been said that necessity is the mother of imaginative creativity. When a great need explodes within someone, it is quite obvious that for that person a definite plan of action must be set up—*immediately*.

As I mentioned earlier, my own personal health was once in great jeopardy. My condition was deteriorating so badly that I was compelled to carry out a plan of heroic proportions, on which I based a new daily ritual. Once my doctor had informed

me that I was stricken with *degenerative rheumatoid arthritis*—
a physical impairment from which I could "never recover"—
it was time for a whole new way of life.

Something had to be done, something that would have to
be accomplished in the least possible amount of time. Precisely
what my program of better living will do for you I haven't the
slightest idea. It is my individual way of using the nine magic
secrets. I want to make crystal clear that I am not offering my
plan as anything more than a set of guidelines. It is entirely up
to you. Frankly, I have no way of knowing how your particular
body chemistry will react to the "magic" products of nature that
have proved to be of such fantastic help to me. But this one thing
I do know: None of the natural food products I am offering for
your consideration are toxic, or have unpleasant side-effects
when eaten as directed on the label.

THE BETTER HEALTH RITUAL

(1) When I hit the deck in the morning, the first thing I
do is drink one full glass of pure spring water—*no
other water will do*—in which I have squeezed the
juice of one-quarter of a lemon.

(2) I perform a few minutes of leisurely stretching and
tensing exercises.

(3) While my balanced breakfast is being prepared—
and this includes all essential nutrients—I pour myself a small glass of orange juice. To this I add a tablespoon of *pure* chlorophyll.

(4) With my orange juice I eat one tablet of a high potency stress formula; two 400 IU capsules of a good
grade of natural E; two 10,000 IU vitamin A capsules

derived from natural sources, and five comfrey tablets. Now I am ready for breakfast.

(5) When 10 o'clock rolls around, instead of indulging in the time-honored coffee break, I eat one capsule of wild red ginseng.

(6) For luncheon I eat small portions of protein, carbohydrates, a fresh raw, or very slightly-cooked vegetable, and a moderate serving of fresh fruit.

(7) When it is time for the mid-afternoon snack, I eat one more wild red ginseng capsule instead of the traditional cup of coffee.

(8) For the "cocktail hour," I pour myself another glass of juice to which I add a tablespoon of *pure* chlorophyll.

(9) When I have completed my evening meal, I eat two or three natural papaya enzyme tablets.

(10) During all of my meals I sprinkle a few grains of a good grade of lecithin granules on my food, particularly my salad, vegetables, sauces, or gravy of any kind.

(11) Two or three times each day I make it a point to recharge my energy potential by sitting quietly for five or ten minutes to clear my mind of the day's trivia and then I give thanks for my perfect health.

(12) Just before retiring, I take a few minutes to rub down briskly with a large coarse towel. It not only tends to stimulate circulation, but it is greatly relaxing.

Once again I want to remind you that the *better living program* that I worked out for my particular needs worked wonders for me, but I haven't the slightest idea what it will do for you. Obviously, each of us has a different *body chemistry* to appease. How you determine your deficiencies can only be accomplished by trying out the Nine Magic Secrets of Long Life until you learn the right balance for you in order to meet your personal requirements, or you can have a competent doctor prepare elaborate and costly testing procedures.

The plans I have scheduled for myself keep me active and are greatly rewarding to me. At an age when most persons are pushing a rocking chair, I am flying to all parts of the free world to keep important lecture engagements.

THE MAGIC MIXER THAT MAKES EVERYTHING ELSE WORK AND EXTENDS LIFE

Perhaps it will seem quite strange to most readers that such an elementary item as *water* could possibly be so vital a step toward your personal miracle of long life, but with a little close observation you will see the fact emerge in all of its pristine clarity.

Contrary to popular belief, there are umteen varieties of drinking water, ranging all the way from distilled, or completely *dead* fluid, to the deliciously sweet, cool water flowing from a high mountain spring. In between you will find all manner of propaganda *hand-outs* favoring this or that type of treatment, or mis-treatment of our precious and steadily-diminishing supply of pure water.

WHY YOU SHOULD DRINK NATURAL UNTREATED WATER

Since we are primarily concerned here with your life span in relation to your intake of clear, pure fluids, we will sidestep the question of how the public water supply should be treated. We'll forget slanted, or influenced news releases, magazine articles and public pronouncements in which extremely dire consequences are predicted for those who oppose the introduction of certain questionable substances into the public water supply. I have read all of the pros and cons on this subject and I am still not enlightened. Suffice to say that the treatment, or mistreatment of water (according to your point of view) for drinking purposes is still quite debatable. In the meantime, I will use only filtered, or untreated deep-well rock-spring water when it is available.

THE ENERGIZING FACTORS OF WATER

In order to launch our discussion on what you should do, let us begin our study in an area of complete agreement: *Water is essential to the living process.* In fact, it is so vital that should a person lose as little as one-fifth of his body liquids he would be inviting a dangerous situation. When you discover that the human body is almost 70% water, you see you should not pass over this reality of existence too lightly.

In this connection, the human expression can be likened to the boiler that supplies steam for the movement of an engine. All of you, I am sure, are familiar with the glass tube that shows the amount of liquid still available to create steam for power. In the physical body the same need prevails, but unfortunately we are not equipped with an external gauge to indicate our body requirements. We must depend upon common sense to direct our intake—and at this point we get into deep trouble for the very plain reason that this need is too often neglected.

WATER IS THE GREAT CONDUCTOR
OF OUR ELECTRIC FORCES

Let us regard for a moment the purpose of water in *sustaining* life. It should be quite obvious to all readers that our body processes are carried on by means of this useful and important liquid. In various solutions all active functions are maintained. Energy is carried to each living cell, toxic body wastes are conveyed to the excretory organs for disposal. The internal organs of kidneys, liver, and stomach should be provided with water, which activates all of the body processes. In this connection, it serves to prolong your life span. When the intake of water is neglected for any reason, the body cells deteriorate, energy units are dissipated and the life forces are in jeopardy, just as the storage battery in your car would go dead should you fail to keep it adequately filled with pure water.

In the steam engine an indicator is provided; in the storage batter capacity can be readily observed by means of a simple testing device, but in the physical body we must depend upon factors established by research *controls.* These directed studies are invaluable because the several lengthy probes and inquiries into the full nature of the living process has revealed many bonus findings that have proved to be extremely helpful in diagnosis. For example, when a person suddenly begins to drink water 'way beyond normal requirements, the presence of diabetes is indicated, according to medical authorities.

WATER FOR <u>YOUR</u> LIVING MIRACLE

For me to assert with great finality the exact amount of water each person should drink during each twenty-four hour period would be assuming an authority I do not possess. The need changes with each and every individual. Some persons can get along very nicely on as little as *six* eight-ounce glasses of water *every day,* while others require as many as ten or more, depending upon size and weight, or the type of work that one is doing, or the weather. However, it is well to note that an intake of *eight* full glasses of water each and every day is about normal for the average individual. Any indulgence that goes far beyond the usual requirements should cause a person to seek a medical check-up, *fast*.

Every man, woman and child should have a glass of pure, fresh water immediately upon rising. After a night's sleep the system needs flushing, and the only substance that can do the job in keeping with natural law is water — plain unadulterated water. This practice is not only vitally important to the every-day living process, it is an absolute must when you are thinking in terms of a long and vigorous life span.

Our body is a storage battery of electric forces which will not hold a charge nor recharge, revitalize or regenerate essential energy units without water.

During the day each person should partake of at least a few ounces of water every hour. Some ingrowing individuals insist that a cup of coffee or a bottle of carbonated beverage supplies the needed liquid, but this person is kidding himself.

WHEN IN DOUBT — TRY A FILTER

In the event that pure fresh water is not available, or the faucet water in your community leaves a great deal to be desired, it is well to note that there are any number of quite adequate filtering devices on the market. Prices on this type of equipment range all the way from three or four dollars up to expensive, large capacity units. Claims made for these appliances, especially in the household field, include such statements as: "Our activated carbon filter design will remove every trace of chlorine, sulphur, fluoride residues, and disagreeable tastes, to leave the water extra clear and sparkling — just like mountain-fresh water."

If the foregoing assertions are accurate, there is no reason why any of us should go without ample supplies of a *pure* life-sustaining liquid, free of questionable additives, and capable of helping us to maintain our program of better living.

LONG LIFE IS NO JOKE

There are any number of stale quips ready and waiting to pass for keen wit whenever the subject of water is mentioned. All of you are familiar with the fast and evasive retort, "Water! What's that?" or even worse, "It rusts my pipes."

When I started my inquiry into ways and means of attaining the miracle of good health, I began "keeping *book*" on every one of my acquaintance. Before too many years it was all too painfully obvious that persons fond of making wisecracks about water, or any facet of the living process, began dropping off soon after reaching the age of forty, while those who would consider and discuss the topic objectively went on to live twenty-five to thirty years longer, with a few of them still going strong after nearly eighty years of life.

Basically, it is safe to assert with great emphasis that any additive introduced into our drinking water *reduces its effectiveness as a life-sustaining, life-prolonging agency.* Possibly this assertion is rather broad, but when we expand the idea even further and declare that this includes coffee, tea, flavored air bubbles, and medications of any kind, we are stepping on commercial toes, but the facts are unmistakable.

I am fully aware that in making these statements I am going 'way out — but if you want facts, all I can do is trot them out for your inspection.

In the next step aimed at bringing the miracle of long life your way, we will emphasize the fact that water is a fascinating and powerful catalyst — the magic mixer that makes everything else work.

THOUGHTS ABOUT
THE "MAGIC MIXER"

(1) Our bodies need clean, pure, unadulterated water in order to sustain and promote a long life span.

(2) All of the living processes require water for the purpose of moving in solution all of the various chemicals that activate and sustain normal body enterprises such as flushing the kidneys of toxic wastes, aiding digestion and stimulating assimilation of the dynamics contained in the food we eat.

(3) Water is essential to the storing and conservation of the vital energies that perpetuate and prolong the miracle of life.

13

THE TRIUMPH OF
LIVING JOYFULLY

There is an important factor in making the nine magic secrets work for you — your attitude toward life. Our attitudes toward ourselves, our associates, our play and our work can only grow out of a healthy and vigorous mind and body fully activated by all of the nine magic secrets. When we are healthy, we can and should enjoy life and appreciate laughter. It seems generally true that if you laugh more you will live longer.

Laughter can be a leavening agent, a catalyst, or a positive reaction which we ourselves can set in motion, which is potent enough to offset at least some of the needless waste of our body energies.

There is a familiar phrase by Ella Wheeler Wilcox that rings true: "Laugh, and the world laughs with you; — weep, and you weep alone." Try having *fun* with everything you do. Laugh *with* the tasks that confront you each day. Enjoy your tasks to the full. Don't make your fun into work, but try to make your work into fun. One of the best quotes I have encountered in recent years appeared in one of the Sunday newspaper supplements, credited to Mary Pettibone Poole: "He who laughs, *lasts.*" The italics are mine so that some of you fast readers won't miss the point.

LAUGHTER IS
THE BEST MEDICINE

My introduction to *the magic of laughing* in restoring good health and greatly extending the life span came to me from Dr. Katsumi Tukuhisa, formerly director of London's vast General Hospital. When I interviewed Dr. Tukuhisa, he related the story of an unusual experience.

One of the wards under his supervision was filled to capacity with *incurables.* This bothered the good doctor. Every time he entered the ward, the feeling of gloom and depression was so heavy in the air that it would pall his whole day. He realized that there had to be a way to overcome this situation.

One day, and quite by accident, as he was entering the ward, one of the nurses said something that struck him funny — so funny, in fact, that he laughed hilariously. In an instant, the atmosphere changed to one of expectancy. All faces turned toward him for the answer. In a flash he got the message. He continued to laugh uproariously until a big grin spread over most of the faces in the room.

Surprisingly, that day the nurses noted a very real improvement in all of the patients in that ward. This was all the clue the doctor needed. The next morning when he entered the room, he came in laughing. The response was meager, but encouraging. After a moment, he said, quietly, "Hereafter when I enter the room I want all of you to start laughing." This failed to go over too well, but the good doctor insisted. Within a few days, most of the patients were responding and within a week the idea got to be contagious. Everyone was greeting him with a hearty laugh whenever he entered the ward.

With this much encouragement, Dr. Tukuhisa made it a point to visit the ward several times each day. Within a month, the so-called incurable patients were checking out of the hospital, apparently completely "healed." Within two months the ward was down to three patients, but even these three were well along to full recovery.

The doctor was so strongly impressed that he resigned his position to found what is now known world-wide as SEICHO-NO-IE. Strangely enough, the idea is catching on in a most fantastic manner. Chapters of the movement are springing up all over Japan, England and America and Dr. Tukuhisa is hitting the lecture trail *with laughter*.

How much fun and laughter can one person stand? This brings up an interesting point for the very plain reason that up until the time this manuscript was released — for better or worse — no reliable researcher within memory has been able to probe the outer limits of a good, honest laugh. Forced laughter, especially in the beginning, will have its limits, but as practice and attitude improve, so will the quality and value of your laughter.

A "LAUGH RECORD"
PAYS OFF — TWICE

After class one afternoon one of the students in my course in Better Living approached me with the following story: "I know this sounds silly, but in one of your early lectures you told the story of why laughter is the best medicine. This idea struck a familiar chord. I remembered that when I was in high school I had bought a *"laugh record"* because it sounded real *groovy* at the time. So, when I returned home that evening I dug around in my storage closet until I found the old record and brought out my discarded record player. At first the family wasn't very enthusiastic about my suggestion. However, since the dinner hour was slowly turning into a very grim affair — and our health was badly in need of improvement — the meal-time accompaniment was tolerated. It wasn't too long after the first attempt that my family was beginning to laugh with the recording and our home took on a whole new atmosphere. I must admit that your idea proved to be a powerful tonic for all of us."

In another instance, and completely unknown to me, one of my students was head nurse at a well-known convalescent hospital. Unable to find a "laugh record," she asked a teacher acquaintance if she could use her tape recorder to make a copy of something she wanted badly. The request was granted and about a dozen others joined in the taping session. When the head nurse began to play the tape over the intercom before breakfast every morning there were some mild protests at first, but only for a short time. Within a week the hospital took on a brand new aura of happiness and the patients were not only easier to get along with, but their needs and requirements dropped to an astonishingly low level. In fact, the formerly over-worked nurses suddenly found themselves with *happy time* on their hands. When the lady reported to me what had happened, she triumphly announced, "And we now have a waiting list of men and women who want to move in with us — and all because our place is so pleasant."

"And how about an improvement in health?" I asked.

"Wow!" was her response. "Everybody but our three bedridden patients are now up and around enjoying life to the limit. The sun room is filled every afternoon with happy people."

Billie Waters of Seal Beach, California, has an infectious laughing problem. "Ever since I can remember," she explained, I was punished for laughing at the wrong time."

Perhaps this natural impulse could be disconcerting to some persons, but she confided "I never have an ache or a pain," and best of all, as I observed, this delightful personality is willing to share her gift of laughter at any time. One of her pet projects is to drop in on convalescent wards where patients are recovering from all manner of infirmaties. She helps such patients learn to laugh. The results of these visits have been little short of spectacular.

The story of Billie Waters was brought to me by Bessie G., vacationing here to escape the cold blasts of a North Dakota winter.

It seems that Bessie suffered a broken hip in one of those crazy household accidents. It was while she was on the mend that she got caught up in the whirlwind of laughter brought on by Mrs. Waters during her frequent visits to the hospital. Soon that laughing at anything and everything got to be a habit. Within a short time Bessie was able to leave the hospital completely mended because of her new attitude — something new and wonderful had been added — laughter. "For years," she told me, "the excruciating pain of arthritis had been creeping up on me to the point where nothing seemed to help. I was soon aware that with my new-found gift of laughter the pain in my joints was getting less almost by the day. It is now six months since I left the hospital and I feel like a new person. In fact, all of the little upsets that come to persons in their senior years no longer bother me one bit. And I owe it all to the fact that I learned to laugh."

A number of people actually pay Billie Waters for her

apparently spontaneous outbursts of laughter. She is hired to add touches of "comedy relief" to some of those home parties that otherwise might get quite dull. But the greatest reward of all comes to her when she is invited to visit hospital wards where laughter is so badly needed.

"Occasionally in home party situations I am called upon to play a clumsy maid who has this laughing problem," she said. "Instead of being apologetic, every time I drop something or do something outrageously wrong, I laugh."

To illustrate her point, Mrs. Waters threw back her head and let go a resounding laugh. She stopped just as suddenly as she began. "That," she said, "is what professional laughers do. They laugh on cue."

FUN MUST HAVE LIMITATIONS

One of the important essentials of fun, either in work or play, stems from a very controversial point — *limited usage.* Fun does not need to be strenuous. I am fully aware that all-day binges in golf, tennis, swimming, in fact, all participation in sports, have many earnest advocates and sponsors. However, I, personally, am overwhelmingly in favor of *short daily periods of activity.*

Just how long is "short" could be debatable, but consensus seems to lean toward periods of indulgence that are limited to fifteen minutes *or less,* with a preponderance of opinion heavily supporting the view that the time to taper off is when the first free flow of perspiration is in evidence.

My objections to the strenuous life could develop into a matter of fiery invective. Many people may object to my alledgedly venturesome ideas, but truth is truth insofar as my position relates to the joyous adventure of extending the life span.

THE IDEAL WORK DAY

Within this same connotation, I am going to advance another belief that is now being borne out of practical realities: The five-hour working day is not only an essential to conserving your resources of energy, *it is a must*.

Entirely aside from the demands of labor leaders, based as they are upon the whims and caprice of the moment rather than upon the economics of supply and demand, there is an even more fundamental and valid reason for supporting the acceptance of this presently controversial issue. *To sustain and prolong the magic of long life, no individual should be required to work* longer than five hours each day, with two full days each week when no work at all is to be done. In practice this would quickly absorb all persons who wanted to be employed; it would greatly increase your reserve of energies.

HOW EXPERIENCE VALUES
CAN BE GREATLY EXTENDED

In addition to the foregoing skills, techniques, and knowledge, together with the perspective that can only come with years of experience, the individual could retain and continue to be active for thirty, forty, even fifty years longer than it is with our presently wantonly extravagant waste of our physical energies.

When this idea is accepted by management, our resources of wealth will be extended so fantastically that by present standards, the results would be considered too imaginative.

The only drawback with this concept stems from a very simple *fact of life* in human nature. *What to do with the extra time?* This query is completely valid, and it is absolutely essential that we have a forthright program ready for action once this great step into the future, of a five-hour working day, is properly activated.

To begin with, one of the greatest needs of our time is adequate in-plant training programs, designed to meet the needs of tomorrow. With the day's work completed, all interested persons could attend classes within the area of company requirements. These groups should be headed by pracitcal persons, skilled in the essentials of developing work needs. Once in awhile a college professor could be brought in with his "way-out" theories and postulates for the sole purpose of keeping attitudes and objectives on the far horizons.

You readers can justly ask a most legitimate question. What does all of this have to do with what we have called *fun?* I fully realize that on the surface this could appear to be quite odd, but in truth we will not be able to slow down the waste of human energies that apparently permeate nearly all of our work activities. It seems so trite and hackneyed to say this, but there is simply too much "gimme" and not enough "give."

WHEN YOU GET YOURS — YOU LOSE

At the present time the attitude is all too prevalent that says in effect, "As long as I get mine, I don't give a damn what happens to you." Well, *that isn't fun,* by a long shot — when you stop to count the cost in creating the magic of long life for yourself, the price you pay is fantastic. This primitive, atavistic, almost stupid indulgence drains off so much of life that it is grotesquely pathetic in its infantilism.

To put it more bluntly, loafing under so-called "make work" rules is not only lavish in the expenditure of life-sustaining forces, it is also destructive to the human spirit. With this illusory benefit goes all respect for law, order, civic responsibility and spiritual values.

DANGER IN "SOCIAL DIVERSIONS"

If, in the foregoing paragraphs I have stepped on some pedal extremities, the yowl that you will hear after reading the next few observations will be as nothing in comparison.

I will say that most long-drawn-out-social-diversions are nothing more than suicidal binges, delightful and a palliative no doubt, but nonetheless self-destructive. For example, a full evening of square dancing with its happy and colorful abandon can cost as much as ten full units of energy, or the potential of *twenty days of life-expectancy*. Quite an exorbitant price to pay for alleged recreation!

An evening of bowling is another excessive and intemperate indulgence. Five person of my acquaintance have dropped dead during long-drawn-out sessions. I am all for this particular sport, but when I play, one game, it is the full extent of my participation — for with one game I am restored and revitalized.

The gist of the idea I am trying to put across here is simply this: Should you want to conserve your energy and create magic in your life, try playing *one game only* of your favorite sport, take part in a single square dance routine, or other recreational activity and let it go at that. Spend the rest of your free time absorbed in reading a good book related to your work or special interests. You will be amazed with the improvement in your health, your work attitude, your family relationships, and a tremendously expanded miracle of healthful living.

DANGER IN ENTERTAINMENT

There are other depleting endeavors that sop up energy units like a dry sponge, but probably the worst malfactor of them all is a grim psycho or horror type movie or TV program. This might seem to be an old-fashioned idea on the face of it, so all I ask you to do is check me out. Observe any person closely who has subjected himself to one of these brutal, mind-devouring sessions. Almost invariably the remark will be made at the close of such a perverted exhibition as, "I feel as if I had been put through a wringer." The fact is, the statement was completely true — with the energies *squeezed* out of them amounting to as much as a full month of life. An inordinate price to pay for so-called fun, or entertainment.

Without any doubt, health, wealth, success, happiness and fulfillment has its origin in a happy mind. Entirely apart from any psychological connotation, *mind* is the source of all of the good things in life. Hence, if we would live long and fruitful lives, we must first cleanse the mind of all that is unworthy before we can begin to draw upon the unlimited energies that are part of our natural heritage.

In *mind*, there are certain steps that must be activated fully before the nine magic secrets of a long life can be made a part of your life expression. These are:

ELIMINATE ALL NEGATIVES
ACHIEVE A MATURE MIND
RELEASE THE PAST
ACCEPT ONLY THAT WHICH IS GOOD
BEGIN NOW TO ACTIVATE THE ENCHANT-
  ING CATALYST OF FUN

Let us now take each of the foregoing points and probe them for realities. To begin with, we will grant that the process of incorporating each of the *directional signals* into your life pattern will be closely akin to swallowing a good old-fashioned dose of caster oil, but, believe me, the effort is well worth the price.

HOW YOU CAN ELIMINATE ALL NEGATIVE EMOTIONS

This, we know, will take some doing. For thousands of years a grim, foreboding attitude has been so much a part of our early training that to change or remove these precious *leftovers* from our consciousness, will require almost a mental cataclysm, but it can be done — and you are the one and only person who can do the job successfully. You can study with competent teachers, attend challenging lectures, go hear *enlightened* ministers every Sunday, but if you fail to take the one most important step of *cleansing your mind,* you will still fall far short of the magic of a longer life.

Whenever I lecture on this subject I always tell the amazing story of June B. For years she would inevitably appear in the front row of my "Better Living" class at the Institute of Lifetime Learning. She was always attentive, always cooperative, until one day she exploded in a most startling manner. "Mr. Hill," she almost barked, "I have been attending your classes for years. I follow my doctor's instructions to the letter. I take my vitamins regularly and I try to follow all of the ideas you suggest for better living, but I am not getting any better. Do you have any idea of what my problem might be?"

For once my intuition was able to meet the challenge! "Who is it you dislike or resent so intensely?" I asked.

For a moment a total look of frustrated amazement swept over Mrs. B's face and then she almost shouted, "My son-in-law! The way he treats me is terrible. I hate his guts!" And with that outburst she subsided almost as if a great pressure had been released.

"All right," I responded, "let's examine the problem with a brief repeat of my lecture covering the topic of *negatives.*"

Obviously, she appeared to be completely bewildered and then a great smile of illumination swept over her face. "Okay," she declared, "from this moment on I am going to love the guy like he's never been loved before. I'm going to bless him a hundred times a day. No matter what he does, I'm going to turn the other cheek. In fact, I'm going to be sweetness and light herself." And with that she flounced out of the room, seemingly too embarrassed to face her peers.

I couldn't help but look forward to the next class session to hear Mrs. B's report. However, she evidently had found her "magic answer" and didn't return to class. It wasn't until nearly a year later that I chanced to meet her on the street. The change in her was nothing less than miraculous. She was absolutely radiant. She was bubbling over with a new zest for life and her first words were, "How can I ever thank you? Believe it or not, my son-in-law and I are now great buddies. I realize now what you meant when you said, *fun is the catalyst.* Everything is working good for me now." With that, she was off to keep an appointment, but showed considerable suppressed excitement.

LIFE AND ENERGY DESTROYERS
YOU CAN ELIMINATE

On the chance that you might not be fully aware of exactly what I mean by *negative,* let us examine a few of the *stand-outs* so that we will be thinking in an area of common agreement.

A "negative" can mean plenty of different things, but for the purpose of our discussion here we will list the ten most virulent of the life and energy destroyers:

(1) *HATES,* even dislikes, when they are strongly expressed are energy consumers.

(2) *FEARS* take a heavy toll of the life forces. Fear of anything — death, taxes, tomorrow, what-others-or-God will think — all of these anxieties, will drain away *wastefully* your needed energies.

(3) *RESENTMENTS, of any kind:* personal slights, real or fancied wrongs, an unhappy turn of events, an apparent adverse *twist of fate,* or luck — all of these things tend to sap a person's vitality if they are accepted and nurtured.

(4) *SUPERSTITIONS* of any kind, regardless of source, have a most depleting effect upon our energies. Eliminate them — *now.*

(5) *SELF-DENIAL* is a needless brake upon the consciousness of man. A really mature mind needs no such imitation discipline.

(6) *PENANCE* is nothing more than a means of accentuating the negative — a measure designed to impress the subconscious mind with failure to the point where deterioration sets in.

(7) *STUBBORNNESS*, or better yet, just plain unadorned *mulishness* will get you nowhere but down. Keep the mind and the cooperative spirit open and receptive at all times. This doesn't mean that you have to go along with every idea that comes your way, or totally adopt all of the suggestions that are presented to you, but at least learn to *weigh and evaluate*. You might gain something — and you will certainly add many more enjoyable years to your life.

(8) *HABITS* are nothing more than repetitive actions, good or bad, that have worn *grooves* in our way of life, and grooves lead in only one direction. When you can change a habit and make your environment more interesting and exciting and full of fun, you have opened up a whole new way of life — and living.

(9) Even *WORK* can be negative when your work isn't stimulating — a real challenge — it is costing you *units* of energy every day. Grow to love what you are doing or else plan to change, improve, or expand your work beginning today — and do it joyfully. This does not mean that you should do something rash or foolhardy, but it does mean to *raise your sights*. The excitement of planning will serve to slow down the spending of energy units.

(10) *POVERTY*. This unnatural situation has to be accepted in mind before it can become real. The condition of poverty is contrary to natural, or Divine Law. It is devastating, demoralizing and spiritually wrong. It can only drain, deplete

and lessen the life forces. Begin now to raise your level of consciousness to a plateau of abundance.

ACHIEVING A MATURE MIND

When we reach the point in *consciousness,* where we can take, and understand, the *measure* of maturity, we will have taken a giant step toward achieving "the maturity concept." In my myriad conversations with persons of good educational background — with men and women who seemed to lead balanced, productive lives — I found all too often that this *concept* was lacking.

In order to bring our search for this *key* to the delightful magic of long life more clearly into focus, we will examine the five *storm signals* that will nearly always indicate the presence of a mind that has failed to grow, no matter how many *previous* accomplishments are in the record. The very minute a person ceases to expand his horizons, he becomes a "has-been" and an energy *leak* has been opened up that can eventually *drain away* all of the body energies.

For a good, honest look at your present *state of mind,* ask yourself for a forthright answer to the following five questions. It is quite important that you come up with an honest evaluation for the very plain reason that there is no one to fool or mislead but yourself.

(1) *Am I defensive?* In other words, do I consistently shirk little responsibilities or obligations and then have to dig furiously to find some plausible explanation for my failure, or am I constantly trying to justify my lack, or incompetency, because of personal shortcomings I have accepted for no good

reason other than to keep me always supplied with an excuse for my faltering performance?

(2) *Temper?* Do I indulge the expensive luxury of *exploding* quantities of my precious energy units by getting childishly emotional over the actions of other persons, an unhappy turn of events, or upsetting accidents in the home or at work?

(3) *Can I "roll with the punches"?* When the adverse twists and turns of fate aim a knockout blow at me, do I take the blow fate gives and let it roll past me with courage, initiative and positive meditation, or do I foolishly step forward, *my chin out,* to receive the full force of the disaster?

(4) *Is my attention toward sex mature?* Better examine this question carefully. Should your *pose* be repressive, it can drain off just as many energy units as if you were overly indulgent and just as much of an obstacle to the attainment of a mature mind.

(5) *Am I always looking backward?* The worst feature of this tendency is that it creates a feeling of *dependence* upon the past. Nearly all of us are familiar with the urge to attend "old grad" rallies. While all of this is often very enjoyable, it can be a great waste of energy units and quite *devitalizing.* Your chief concern should be with *today* and the days to come with the ever-growing promise of fulfillment.

HOW YOU CAN RELEASE THE PAST AND REVITALIZE AND REGENERATE YOUR FUTURE

Whoever said, "revenge is sweet," was not only a knothead, but a wastrel of no mean attainments. The very idea of *vengeance* might placate the ego of an immature person; however, it should be known to the man or woman indulging in this costly palliative that with every twinge of hate, there is dissipated a flood of *energy units* that cannot be replaced too easily. Hate, bitterness or malevolence not only shrivels the soul, but this feeling of wanting to bring retribution to a person for a real or imagined wrong, has a tendency to *contract*, irrevocably, the capacity to retain, or regenerate, life-extending energy units.

"Let there be peace on earth, and let it begin with me," are the words from a very wonderful song. Take this wisdom to heart. Make it part of your everyday pattern of living. You can make a good beginning this very hour by releasing *all* of the past with its grievances, frustrations, and injustices. Plan to go happily forward into a bright new world of *tomorrow,* all filled to overflowing with *good.* Many additional years of happy, zestful living will be your reward.

WHY YOU SHOULD ACCEPT
ONLY THAT WHICH IS GOOD

Once you have cleansed the mind of *energy-consuming negatives,* it will be possible to *deny* all that is harmful, depleting or worthless. When the first reluctant step is taken, each succeeding forward effort will become easier, until you have surmounted all of the ruinous thinking habits that you have tended so carefully — *even disease.* It might take a little time, but complete *victory* is possible. How long this will be depends upon three things:

(1) The strength of your determination to escape the past.

(2) The intensity of your desire to go forward into a joyous new life.

(3) The depth of your involvement with thinking and living patterns lacking in the use of the catalyst, *fun*.

LET FUN PREVAIL
AT ALL TIMES

James Elmo, writing in *Let's Live* magazine, quotes John Davidson, popular motion picture personality, TV host, and entertainer as saying, "Half of being alive is mental." Davidson is a firm believer in *activity* rather than shadow-boxing with time. According to his interviewer, he is always on the move — with a happy purpose. The philosophy of this famous actor is that to be alive you must act alive *with joy*.

In summing up this particular step to the magic of a long and exciting life, the point I want to emphasize again and again is simply this: enter into all of your activities — and this means work or play — in a spirit of fun. Enjoy everything that you do right up to the hilt, including an irksome chore that you would like very much to avoid. You can, if you try, find something in the unpleasant task to enjoy even though the sole reward is getting it done. This might sound a little far out, but in action this method does save and extend the forces that prolong the magic of long life — YOURS.

THOUGHTS ABOUT
REVITALIZING YOURSELF

(1) Slow down your aging process by developing a forward looking attitude, an attitude of joy.

(2) Plan to grow in a happy consciousness each day by constantly reaching out, for new and thrilling experiences.

(3) Start each day with joyous anticipation, so that the free-flowing channels of cosmic energy can revitalize and regenerate your physical body.

14

LOOK AWAY, LOOK AWAY
TO A LONG AND REWARDING LIFE

Since it is well known in science that *a body at rest tends to remain at rest,* our chief problem is how to overcome this natural inertia that serves to shorten life.

"Where to start?" is the sticky morass that captures and holds all too many of us in the gummy clutches of senility. It is to escape this plague of humankind that I will supply you with the one-word formula that never fails to increase enjoyable years of good living. It is *movement,* any kind of movement. For the outstanding trait of character that must be cultivated is to constantly be on the alert to *start something.* And by this I obviously mean any course of action that could eventually be helpful, revealing, or profitable.

Perceptive observation is the essential KEY to developing movement *and eventual attainment* of a goal in this area of speculative venturing. And in addition there must be a close evaluation of *what happens* when you do hazard the raised eyebrows of your contemporaries by daring to lift the lid of possible creative action. I can only urgently suggest that you keep a notebook or a note pad handy *and take the time to record every step, change, development or result of the thing you are attempting.*

HERE ARE SOME THINGS TO TRY OR ATTEMPT:

(1) LOOK OVER THE FENCE. Just for practice, look into the so-called "green pastures" of activities different from the ones you cherish. Select any likely idea that comes to your attention and translate the plan, the process or the procedure into terms and methods friendly to your way of life. It is always possible that the course of action you are *trying* could turn your life style into one of rewarding adventure.

(2) ALWAYS BE CURIOUS. Whenever you can, read, read, read! It could be newspapers, business or professional trade papers, publications — or, better yet, subscribe to these specialized periodicals. I have always found them to be loaded with ideas for venturing.

(3) TAKE "FIELD TRIPS." Take the *eye-opening* time to visit plants, factories or special types of leisure time opportunities, especially those different from your own. The experience is not only good for enlarging background values, it is also tremendously helpful in stimulating the creative processes of your mind.

(4) KICK YOUR QUESTIONABLE HABITS INTO REVERSE. In your own way of life take your hoary *tried and true* routines and one by one try doing them differently.

(5) TRY "LEFT FIELD." When you have exhausted all other possibilities, boot your customary way of doing things completely *out of bounds* and into a new area of activity. This can usually be achieved by putting your old habits on ice for a day. This practice in action has often created some new and exciting life styles, and especially has it served to scrap old practices in a most delightful manner.

(6) LOOK IN THE FUN HOUSE MIRROR. This idea has been tried mostly for laughs, but it has produced some rather startling results. In your own life pattern, take any one of your daily routines and try looking in a mirror that will distort your fixed ways — or try creating a silly invention for the purpose of performing your well established habit in the style of Rube Goldberg.

(7) BE A "COPY CAT." Let me remind you of a basic fact in the art of creativity: "That man is most original who can adapt from the greatest number of sources." Whenever you encounter an idea that some enterprising man or woman has used to change an old habit, apply the plan mentally to your own situation. The concept that is born of this combination of ideas could mean the difference between an average dull person and a rewarding way of life.

GREAT MINDS OF THE PAST
ARE FULL OF TREASURE

In our personal thinking, we should first learn to take advantage of the great minds of the past. It is regrettable that so many of us are continually trying to find some new idea, some special formula, or even a magic key, that will enable us to achieve a long and happy life. For a moment let us regard the words of Goethe, who offered this sage advice in a rare moment of perception: "All truly wise thoughts have been thought already thousands of times. To make them truly ours we must think them over again honestly *until they take root in our experiences.*"

EACH NEW LEVEL OF CONSCIOUSNESS IS VALUABLE

Just as there are many planes of experience, so is it true that there are many levels of thinking, and the grade or value of our *thought power* is exactly equal to our present *level of consciousness.* To explain this phrase in relation to the idea of holding back the years, we must go back and examine again the ingredients that support a high plateau of genuine awareness.

Since it is known that "thoughts are things," it goes almost without saying that each thought has a definite value. It is more than obvious that we are on one level of thought when we are considering our needs in matters of health, success, or happiness, and quite another when we go on to regard the greater values that contribute an idea or a thought toward our own better living program.

Each level of thought has its own ground rules for thinking, regardless of whether it is frivolous, scattered, or unrelated, or if the full power of thought is invoked with directed, organized and purposeful attention. Therefore it is plain that each type of thought requires its own degree of concentration. To begin our progress toward all of the good that life has to offer, each of us can implement our plan of growth by training ourselves to think, with *concentration,* about the ordinary problems of the day. When we have organized our *thought processes* to the point where we can meet and solve the issues of today, then we are ready to go on to ever higher levels of thought wherein the riches of true happiness, fulfillment and long life are stored.

THE KEY TO LONG LIFE

Actually, the most important value I ever gained from reading books covering the subject of auto-suggestion was the basic formula for using the boundless power of affirmation for personal growth, but I will admit that it took some digging to finally isolate the relevant words and phrases and to translate them into as understandable sequence. Here it is:

> To achieve what you want, be it health, long life, great wealth or recognition, you must *want* strongly enough, with all of the might of your being, to achieve, or to be healed.

Right this very minute you can start a prairie fire of increased vitality that will sweep you to any height of physical vigor that you select. The choosing is up to you, but you should begin now to light up your pathway by striking off many new creative sparks today.

COLLECTING VALID HEALTH IDEAS

In a bygone century, a dour old Scotsman by the name of Thomas Carlyle struck off a flinty thought when he declared: "That man is most original who can adapt from the greatest number of sources." You probably have discovered that that quotation is one of my favorites and I use it many times. In other words, all you have to do is start to collect valid health ideas wherever you find them. When you have accumulated a smart assortment of thoughts, plans, designs, or even devices, regardless of whether they are related or not, and begin to use them cautiously in any combination that pleases your fancy, you will have claimed the first easy steps to a long and rewarding way of life.

At this point it is important that you understand the exact nature of *creative thinking*. To bring this concept into clear focus for future references, I suggest a well-known quote from *The Mature Mind,* by H. A. Overstreet:

"Imagination is making new wholes out of familiar parts."

When our prehistoric ancestors got an idea, they acted upon it, often impulsively. Naturally enough, they got results, not always what they wanted, but things did happen. It was in this rather haphazard manner that a vast source of experience values began to grow. Think what you can do with 10,000 years of background information to draw upon. And so it is that we open the door for you to a bright new future, with *imagination* providing the magic key to an exciting way of life.

Once the highly energized forces of the imagination have been sparked into action, the next vitally important step is to *condition the mind to accept good health*. On the face of it this might seem to be a needless precaution, but the truth of the matter is that the very moment you turn toward a higher level of physical well-being, *things begin to happen*. Once the flood gates of abundant living are opened, it requires all of the limitless powers of the mind in full force to remain calm, poised and *on course,* so great are the dynamic influences of positive thinking.

In a practical sense, for example, the art and science of experimenting has two important aspects. These are: (1) To prove an already known Law of Nature; (2) To discover an unknown, but suspected, Law of Nature. Consequently, the aim, the intent, and the purpose of *experimenting* with your new way of life is either proof or discovery.

As I have previously explained, in the beginning of time our pre-historic ancestors got an idea and with little thought or planning acted upon his or her inspiration. Invariably something happened. The results were not always exactly welcome, but something new was added to the slowly expanding scope of knowledge. And so it was in this manner that a vast amount of experience-values began to grow.

Once again, stop and think for a moment about this startling fact: "What I can do with 10,000 years of background information to draw upon is without limit."

YOUR OWN TREMENDOUS
DATA PROCESSING DEVICE

In a more practical way, memory is a storehouse of information. It can be compared to the most expensive and elaborate piece of data processing equipment ever devised. The only difference is that the human memory possesses a capacity and flexibility that is without limit. Facts, impressions, data, pictures, even statistics, are fed into memory, first by observation and experience, then it is extended by the process of formal education.

The attribute of memory is a many splendored, many faceted potential of the normal human equation. The full extent of this great power has never been fully explored.

It is true that this faculty of mind has inspired endless discussion throughout the ages. It has been the subject of interminable lectures, courses of study and an impressive array of booklets, all purporting to give the reader an *open sesame* to the wonders of retaining and reviving impressions, or how best to recall and use previous experiences.

Actually, the ability *to remember* is based upon five equally important activities. To neglect any one of them is to lessen the quality of this perceptive power of mind. They are:

(1) Attention
(2) Interest
(3) Association
(4) Concentration
(5) Review

According to Thomas Mann, the control tower affecting your destiny is in your head: "Human reason needs only to *will* more strongly than fate, and she *is* fate."

The apparently endless debate over the full meaning of *freedom of will* seems to have a tendency to tower over the theory of the will itself. Actually, when this great principle of mind power is reduced to an understandable sentence, the meaning and intent of *will* is quite clear: *Each of us possesses a built-in guidance system.*

The only catch to this obviously ingenuous explanation appears to erupt from the fact that this powerful directional force must be trained. And the only person in the whole wide universe who can activate this program of personal management is *you*. Will, or *will power* is an attribute that must be cultivated. There is no other way to master this immense, energized force.

When a person fails to assume command of this action *governor,* the results are inevitably negative, and often chaotic.

The lack of personal initiative in actively taking over the office of *director* of will power has made mediocre, or worse, has destroyed, all too many promising persons. Let us know that this will not happen to you.

The difference between the "right action" and *"almost* the right action" to paraphrase a Mark Twain observation, "is the difference between lightning and the lightning bug."

For example, the original intent of speech was to make known the elementary needs of self-preservation. Moreover, this transfer of ideas was limited to mere grunts that were bandied about with varying degrees of emphasis in order to convey meaning. With the passage of time — many thousands of years in fact — these harsh sounds evolved into words with a single meaning and purpose.

THE REAL VALUE OF
HUMAN COMMUNICATION

In the beginning a limited vocabulary served the needs of prehistoric man, but eventually a steadily increasing population brought with it, through scattered generations, a few new terms. True enough, these original improvements in speech were quite simple. In fact, even now the ability to communicate with one another is so fundamental to the human concept that its real values are often lost upon most persons. In this connotation, the idea of conveying thought by simply talking has been overworked to the point where the real meaning of this faculty seems to get a trifle fuzzy at times.

The real reason why ideas, instructions or directions break down between individuals, or even associates, quite often derives from the fact that someone wasn't *listening*. This situation prevails in all three methods of transmitting any type of information. Why this should be true is a paradox that is difficult to understand, since the faculty of hearing is common to nearly all persons. Obviously then, it is the very ease with which listening is accomplished that makes it an arduous task.

First of all, we know that opportunities for better living never cease to literally hammer on the door of any person willing to listen. Not only can it offer a golden chance to increase your experience without the expenditure of additional time, money or effort, but it can also add greatly to your enjoyable years.

For example, back in the early, experimental years of psychological research, some intrepid, questing investigator attached the prefix *sub* to the vast realms of the *unknown mind*. Apparently this term derived from the fact that knowledge, once acquired, seemed to sink under the conscious level of thinking, and was therefore below the normal range of the intellect.

As the human expression grew in awareness, there was an ever-expanding tendency to return to the concepts of mind that were enunciated when the Supreme Intelligence created man *in His own image,* and decreed that he should hold dominion over the earth. It never ceases to amaze me that the most important part of this pronouncement is neglected, or worse, relegated to a lesser place in all but the cloistered halls of remote philosophical or theological centers. It is this: *Man must first learn to manage, control, and thus conquer himself.*

Since the creative potential of the *sub* or supra conscious mind is without limit, it naturally follows that *feeding* this sensitive extension of the conscious mind should be carefully regulated. That is, learning interests, reading habits, experience values, study routines, research objectives, and imagination should be kept well within the confines of a single purpose.

APPLYING YOUR INNER POWERS

Once more, I want to remind you that the mind is far superior to any assembled piece of data processing equipment yet devised. It can be activated and made useful so easily that its value escapes most persons. To attempt to impart a reasonable concept of the full potential of this natural endowment by means of ordinary similes is difficult, but I will use the following comparison: *If you multiply your present capabilities by 10,000, you will have a rough idea of the power and magnitude of your supra conscious mind.*

With the foregoing fact firmly in mind, it is easy to understand why each and every *mental movement* should be gently but resolutely directed in one positive direction — first to acquire as much general or foundation knowledge as possible, and second to guide attitudes, energies, and interests toward your objective.

In the beginning there will be problems to solve, obstacles to overcome and frustrations to surmount. It is how you resolve these intermediate issues that will determine how successful you will be when you come face-to-face with major health problems that must be managed to personal advantage.

THOUGHTS ABOUT MAKING THE MOST OF THE NINE MAGIC SECRETS

(1) To achieve a long and rewarding life, the KEY WORD is *movement.*

(2) Affirm with great determination: "I will eagerly, and

with great zeal, put real life into the seven basic rules of *movement.*"

(3) Know that with each new level of positive consciousness you will attain will add years to enjoyable living.

(4) Recognize and *accept* the fact that wanting something worthy and with great intensity is one of the basic elements that serve to support the *Nine Magic Secrets of Long Life.*

(5) Understand that a lively and active imagination is the catalyst that serves to put fire-power into your quest for a long, happy and rewarding life.

YOUR LONG LIFE POTENTIAL

When Walter Pitkin, best-selling author of a generation past, first enunciated the theory that each of us is born with X number of energy units, he managed to stir up quite a *rukus* in the scientific community — especially when he went on to declare that when you have exhausted your personal supply your life is ended.

At the time his belief was met with open incredulity, often outright derision. However, time and the tides of research are now in full support of his *way out* concept. To translate this abstraction into easily understood terms, it means that you have approximately two energy units to use every day in order to reach the biblical pronouncement of *"three-score-and-ten" years.*

How this temperate use of energy units is accomplished is entirely a personal matter. You can waste the life-sustaining store of energy units with prodigal abandon, or you can husband them. Obviously, if you could spend only one unit each day you could reasonably extend your life span to *one hundred and forty years.*

How you can accomplish this desired end will now be revealed to you — in terms that you can understand.

To begin with you should know that we spend from eight to ten energy units in performing our day's work. Without replenishing your natural heritage with the regenerative factors I have made known to you, you would probably live less than a year. The restorative elements you should use have all been explained to you with the exception of sex. Contrary to popular religious beliefs, sex is three-fold in purpose instead of one. They are: procreation, recreation and *regeneration.* Within the latter frame of reference, sex, when used properly between male and female, equal and opposite to each other, positive and negative poles of reaction, energy units can be restored in a most fantastic manner. How this is achieved is a subject for a completely new discussion.

YOUR LONG LIFE POTENTIAL TEST

On a scrap of notepaper, jot down your honest answers to this test. When you can truthfully answer "YES" to the following questions you can reasonably expect to *double* your life expectancy.

(1) Are you married to a congenial and fully cooperative person?

(2) Are you less than 10% underweight or overweight?

(3) Do you make certain your blood pressure is within normal limits?

(4) Do you eat only raw or slightly cooked foods?

(5) Have you stopped smoking?

(6) Do you avoid eating processed foods of any kind?

(7) Do you carefully avoid ALL of the five deadly whites in your daily intake of food?

(8) Do you take a few minutes every day to invoke the POWER OF BREATH with deep breathing exercises?

(9) Do you drink enough pure spring water every day in order to supply minimum body requirements?

(10) Do you make it a point to stretch and tense gently at least twice each day?

(11) Do you indulge in a good hearty laugh several times each day?

(12) Do you spend a few relaxing minutes each day with a vibrating pad, chair, or table?

(13) Do you supplement your daily intake of food with a natural vitamin-mineral combination?

(14) Do you include one or more natural enzyme tablets after each meal according to your particular body requirements?

(15) Have you developed *your own* BETTER LIVING PROGRAM, keeping in mind always your own body requirements?

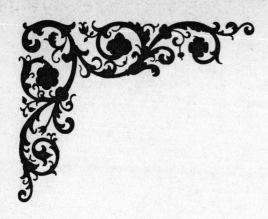

SOURCES OF
BASIC BUILDING BLOCK FOODS

ENZYMES. This valuable natural food derives from the fruit of the papaya tree. It is known as the "magic melon of the tropics." The greatest claim to fame of the papaya enzyme is its uncanny ability to aid in the digestion of foods, especially proteins. Nearly all health food stores carry this product in one form or another, but the one I have found most reliable is a product of Tested Natural Organics, a Division of Universal Nutrition, Inc., Yonkers, N. Y. 10703.

CHLOROPHYLL. Once again there are numerous varities of this highly versatile product, many of them with so many additives that the "green magic" can no longer be classed

as natural. The two versions of the liquid I prefer are processed
by Paul de Sousa's company, P. O. Box 1144, San Jacinto, Calif.
92383, or the Organic Sea Products Corporation, Burlingame,
Calif. 94010.

COMFREY. Many reliable firms are now turning out
Comfrey tabs in ever increasing quantities, but the one that
seems to be the most reliable is produced by Essential Foods
Co. Inc., Milwaukee, Wisconsin, 53233. The company claims
the tablet form is produced by a special cold process from
powdered and defibered comfrey leaves grown on the controlled farms of the firm.

LECITHIN. This amazing yield of the lowly soybean is
well known in over a thousand manufacturing processes because of its ability to emulsify. In the human body it has a well
deserved reputation for dissolving the "crud" that causes hardening of the arteries. Many arthritic sufferers report relief from
painful formations. It is available in both capsules and granules
in any health food store.

SPROUTS. Should you be aware of the healthful qualities
of sprouts, or the nutritional values of the seeds from which
they grow, you can become an expert in their cultivation very
easily. For full instructions write to Jolley's, P. O. Box 145,
La Mirada, Calif. 90638. These tasty bits of emerging plant life
are loaded with food values of great merit.

GINSENG. The root of the ginseng plant has been a staple
in the bag of tricks of herb doctors for many centuries. So many
claims have been made for this oddly shaped tuber that one's
credulity is stretched — way out. Most persons prefer the powdered root in capsule form. However, it is well to be wary.
Should you want to try ginseng it is better to seek out a reliable
health food store, one that stocks only guaranteed products.

VITAMIN E. As this is being written this amazing product derived from quality grains is available from a multitude of sources. Most health food stores carry this item in all potencies. Many super markets maintain a vitamin shelf, and nearly all of the major direct selling companies carry Vitamin E in both tablet and capsule form, with the latter greatly favored because the oil can be used for the relief of some skin problems.

INDEX